Surviving Type II Diabetes

(In Spite of the Experts' Advice)

by

Dr. Rick Boatright

Bloomington, IN  Milton Keynes, UK

authorHOUSE™

AuthorHouse™
1663 Liberty Drive, Suite 200
Bloomington, IN 47403
www.authorhouse.com
Phone: 1-800-839-8640

AuthorHouse™ UK Ltd.
500 Avebury Boulevard
Central Milton Keynes, MK9 2BE
www.authorhouse.co.uk
Phone: 08001974150

First published by AuthorHouse 4/12/2006

ISBN: 1-4259-2316-X (e)
ISBN: 1-4259-2315-1 (sc)

Library of Congress Control Number: 2006902198

Printed in the United States of America
Bloomington, Indiana

This book is printed on acid-free paper.

This book is dedicated to my lovely wife, Linda McBride-Boatright, without whose love, encouragement, gentle guidance, long hours of editing and scientific diligence, this book would never have developed.

Contents

Forward

Many centuries ago, a diligent and observant young man made some revolutionary conclusions based on the conjecture of a few heretically observant men before him and on his own personal observations. He had been watching the movements of the sun, moon and stars. However, his conclusions flew in the face of all the conventional wisdom of his day. Anybody with only one eye could plainly see that the sun and the moon always rise in the east and that they always set in the west. No matter where one is on the earth, these heavenly bodies always rise in the east and set in the west, every single day, 365 days a year. Except for some seasonal variations, the periods of darkness when the sun was gone were roughly equivalent to the periods of light. It should be blatantly obvious to anyone who watches the skies, more or less indisputably, that the sun orbits the earth every 24 hours, just as the moon orbits the earth on a regular, predictable schedule. Any fool could see that! All the great thinkers and wise men, every man of learned authority of that time, knew that this was a true and invariable fact that could not be argued.

But now we know that this heretic lunatic with his new and outrageous conclusions wasn't insane at all. Galileo, even though he spent the last years of his life under house arrest for heresy for having the audacity of presenting his revolutionary ideas, went down in history as a man who saw reality from a new perspective – the one that happened to be true. The earth spins on its axis.

Our observations can be quite accurate, very precise and absolutely undisputed such as, "the sun always rises in the east and sets in the west, day after day, year after year." But our conclusions, as obvious as they may seem at first, may be completely wrong, simply because it has never occurred to us to consider other possibilities – erroneous conclusions such as, "…the sun must therefore orbit the earth!"

In the nineteenth century, a man developed a new and revolutionary technology, but when he presented this new idea to the scientific community of his day, they wouldn't even listen to what he had to say. The idea was certainly a complete impossibility and this man must surely be a raving nut, they thought, having lost all of his sense of reason. Instead of humoring him long enough to hear him out or to test his theory, they simply locked him up and tried him for incompetence. When he revealed his preposterous idea in court, it was obvious this poor fellow was out of his mind. He lost his fight and was institutionalized for a year.

You may not be familiar with the name of Antonio Marconi, but you're certainly on intimate terms with the technology he introduced to the world. He was the man who tried to explain to the scientists of his day that he had discovered a way to send audible messages from one location to a distant location without the use of direct wires. He called this strange new technology "radio."

He faced the greatest, wisest, most learned scientists of his day. But because his insights and ideas did not conform to their established parameters, he was considered to be the one with the fundamentally flawed mental processes.

"We've always done it this way" thinking and "this is obviously the way it is" conclusions are the stuff of intellectual stagnation, the quicksand that impedes the progress of truth and mankind's understanding of reality.

Albert Einstein defined insanity as, "Continuing to do the same thing over and over again, expecting a different result."

The true scientist is open to new thoughts, whether they conform to our comfortable, current theories or not. The true scientist never says that a particular thing is impossible, but rather observes the reality before him or her without prejudice. The true scientist refrains from saying, "it can't be" but instead asks "how?"

Any person in the scientific community who thinks that we, in our twenty-first century wisdom, have it all figured out is simply delusional. New scientific studies are published daily that either expand upon or contradict information that we have assumed for years was complete and true. The body of human knowledge changes and expands constantly.

Statistically, if you were to begin reading only the new scientific papers that are published from today on, reading 24 hours a day, 365 days a year, within the first year, you would be about 20 years behind in your reading!

Today's conventional wisdom, the current assumptions of healthcare scientists, hold out certain bits of information to be absolutely true. No doubt. They can be compared to the facts that the sun always rises in the east and always sets in the west, and that the darkness and the light are approximately equal over the course of the year.

But I believe that the healthcare sciences, including their traditional, ancillary nutritional professions, have made some erroneous assumptions about many of those observations, assumptions that I think are as skewed as the assumption that the sun orbits the earth daily.

In this book, you'll see many of the scientific facts that you've read for years, but they'll be put together in ways most of you have not seen before. Many healthcare professionals will disagree with me, clinging to a, "but we've always done it this way," rationale, but other conscientious practitioners are partially responsible for me learning what I'll be presenting in this text. Many of my colleagues in the alternative healthcare professions will also disagree with me on similar grounds. But others will immediately recognize this line of reasoning and the logic of my conclusions. I acknowledge from the beginning that this information contradicts conventional wisdom, but as I've tried to illustrate above, conventional wisdom is not always the complete truth.

Alternative healthcare professionals tried to convince the medical profession for decades that our foods could no longer provide all of the nutrition we need as human beings, only to be rebuffed and derided as "health nuts" who were touting information without scientifically backed merit. However, just in the past few years, the prestigious "Journal of the American Medical Association" published its latest official opinion that every American should supplement with vitamins daily, admitting that this information was 30 years late making it into print in the scientific journals. We're always taking steps forward as we learn more and more. In the process, we must let go of old, outdated ways of thinking.

In all fairness, I can't say with 100% certainty that my conclusions, presented in this book, are the absolute, complete truth either, although I believe they're a step in that direction. I do know that the current conventional wisdom is not working for the majority of my own patients who insist on adhering to those outdated recommendations. I do know that those of my patients, friends and family who have given me feedback about following the information you're about to read have enjoyed success that surpasses the levels being achieved by following today's conventional medical wisdom.

Mrs. M., 64, was diagnosed with type II diabetes in late 2003. As my chiropractic patient, she has closely followed the recommendations outlined in this book ever since. Initially, her blood sugar was approaching 500 mg/dl, a dangerously high level. Without using any drugs, she has now seen her blood sugar under 180, has lost more than 80 pounds, no longer feels the parasthesias (strange sensations) in her hands and feet, heals faster than she has in years, no longer feels crabby so often, has more energy and loses a lot less time at work.

Mr. B., 59, had a blood sugar reading of 285. (Above 180 is considered diabetic.) Following the recommendations in this book, he has dropped his blood sugar to 150, also without drugs. He's dropped 40 pounds, no longer craves sweets, no longer overeats or even wants to, says he's far more patient and is now comfortable with his cholesterol levels.

Mr. E. was diagnosed with type II diabetes long before he became my patient. After many years on medications and enduring their side effects, he asked one day if there were any way he might be able to control his diabetes naturally. I offered only parts of the information in this book, but within just a few months, he had brought his blood sugar under control within the normal range, lost 28 pounds, reduced his food cravings and was enjoying life with a renewed verve.

I know beyond any reasonable doubt that critics of my work will loudly proclaim that it's not backed up by double-blind, scientific studies. And they will be partially correct. Much of it isn't, but a lot of it is. The parts that are not are still, however, backed by clinical observation, in other words, we've tried it, others have tried it, and it produces the desired result in a predictable pattern in clinical application with real live people in real life situations, regardless of whether or not anyone has done "double blind, controlled studies" in a laboratory setting.

My intent in writing this book is not to point out medical shortcomings or to blemish the integrity of the healthcare sciences or anyone within them. I must assume that all of us enter this calling with the highest motives of helping our fellow Souls to achieve and maintain 100% of our maximum health potentials or as close to that as possible. I applaud every human being who espouses such motives.

My intention is only to present currently known information in a different way, to present the same, basic observations but with different conclusions. My assumptions, based on the same scientific building blocks, lead me to a different way of viewing the subject as a whole.

I don't in any way compare myself to the great thinkers like Galileo; however, the concept is similar. He used the same scientific observations as his fellow scientists; the pattern of the sun rising and setting; but put that information together in a new and different way. We've since discovered that he was right – the earth is a revolving orb facing a fixed sun giving us the illusion that the sun is orbiting the earth.

As a legal disclaimer, I must state that the information in this book is not intended as a means of rendering a diagnosis nor does it constitute a prescription for treatment. Rather, it is a report of my own findings, my study of the current science as I understand it, my conclusions based on that science, how I've worked to implement those conclusions and what this entire process leads me to believe is true as a trained, licensed, practicing healthcare practitioner.

I can't advise you to abandon the advice of your doctor, but I can tell you that I bet my own life and my own health on this information as does my wife, Linda. I offer this information to my own patients, with the same disclaimer, so that they can have a second opinion and an alternative way of reasoning through what they hear and read and so that they can make their own, informed decisions about their health.

My voice may be something of a cry in the dark, but it's not mine alone. Others, such as Dr. Robert Atkins, Dr. Michael Eades and Dr. Mary Dan Eades, have cried out before me or I would never have come to my current understanding.

My wife, Linda, is challenged with type II diabetes herself. As a clinical laboratory scientist, she has years of experience working in hospital laboratories in Oregon and Arizona and teaching at Arizona State University. Her clinical laboratory experience has provided much of my inspiration and contributed a great deal of the information that appears in this book.

I hope that as you read this text you'll be able to glean from it specific concepts that you can integrate into your own life, activities that may contribute significantly to your well-being, your true health, your longevity and your quality of life within that longevity.

And, if you would be so kind, if you have any feedback for me about your success with this information or variations on it, please write and let me know in care of the publisher.

Dr. Rick Boatright

Introduction

When my wife and I first discovered that she was a type II diabetic, and that I was on the verge of it myself, she went unwaveringly onto the dietary straight and narrow from that very moment and I was right on her heels. Since my challenge wasn't as severe as hers, I haven't had to be quite as strict, but nonetheless, monitoring my eating habits has certainly proven that I can't stray even slightly without suffering scientifically measurable consequences myself.

Amazingly, even though I had studied both type I and type II diabetes in my training to become a doctor of chiropractic and although my wife, Linda, had performed innumerable hospital laboratory blood tests and understood much of the physiology of both types of diabetes in her career as a clinical laboratory scientist, neither of us truly understood the depth and the true nature of these two, dramatically different types of diabetes until she faced the diagnosis of type II for herself.

Her diagnosis came on the Thanksgiving weekend of 2003. We were entertaining family that weekend. Linda's brother-in-law had been diagnosed some years ago with type II diabetes and he tested his blood regularly to monitor his blood sugar levels. You'll be reading more about the importance of doing this in several places throughout this book. Being a clinical laboratory scientist, Linda had been suspicious for some time that some of her recent health challenges might have been due to high blood sugar levels – one of the symptoms associated with both types of diabetes. So when her brother-in-law brought out his testing meter on November the 29th, she asked if she could use it to test her own blood sugar as well.

The reading she got was very high. In fact, it was high enough to be in a range for which she had seen many people hospitalized during her career as a laboratory scientist. The diagnosis of type II diabetes was indisputable.

We both knew a lot about the harmful role of carbohydrates in type II diabetes, so Linda made a complete shift in her mental concepts and her use of food that very moment. I knew from some recent studies and from the blood glucose meter reading that I saw on myself that day that I was rapidly approaching the same condition. I also knew that the reason I carried so much unwanted weight was due to my body habitually producing inappropriately overabundant amounts of insulin. I had acquired a marked over-sensitivity to carbohydrates, a classic sign of the pre-diabetic condition. I was hungry all the time and got crabby if I missed a meal or if one was more than a half an hour or so past its usual time. I seemed to spend all of my days hanging on the refrigerator door, munching, and would still go to bed not feeling satisfied.

But at the time, our understanding of diabetes was still somewhat fuzzy as we now believe it is for the majority of healthcare professionals. When you find yourself with a condition that can threaten your life and in the meantime make your life very uncomfortable, you have a tendency to dig far deeper to understand as much about it as you can. Losing our feet or our eyesight, common eventualities for diabetics, was something we wanted to avoid at all costs if we could.

What we've learned through our personal research, experimentation and personal experience, backed by my medical training, 20 years of experience as a practicing doctor and annual re-licensing training together with Linda's university training, many years of teaching laboratory sciences to doctors, nurses and other laboratory scientists and more than 20 years as a practicing clinical laboratory scientist herself, has brought us to some startling conclusions. Most importantly, we believe that the majority of "experts" are confused, to say the least, about the differences between the two types of diabetes. In particular, they have a poor and incomplete understanding of the nature of type II diabetes specifically.

In fact, much of the information that is available today about type II diabetes in the popular literature, such as magazine and newspaper articles, in standard healthcare circles, and in the recommendations of professional nutritionists, is actually harmful. This erroneous, albeit popular advice, can contribute to worsening the type II diabetic condition over time because their understanding of what it is and why and how it develops is incomplete. And worse, even though treating type II diabetes with drugs, such as Glucophage, may sometimes lessen some of the symptoms of type II diabetes, it practically guarantees the advancement of the life-threatening effects of the "disease" itself, especially if there are no proven, effective, dietary changes made at the same time. The drugs may manipulate a limited number of symptoms, but they simply do nothing to address the underlying cause of those symptoms.

You'll note that I put the word "disease" in parentheses because type II diabetes is not a true disease such as in the case of type I. As you'll learn later, it's really a complex, physiological, survival adaptation in our bodies, a series of reflexes and long-term training of organs in an effort to protect us from our own self-destructive habits. But even though it's an effective survival strategy in the short run, it's one that runs amok over time.

Until you truly understand this complete process yourself, you'll remain the unwitting victim of self-proclaimed "experts" who may be well-meaning in giving their kind and generous advice, but who are preaching a combination of old wives tales and misinformation, mixing aspects from different diagnoses, and espousing a, "but we've always done it this way," philosophy. People who have followed the recommendations in this book, as a rule, have been able to establish greater control of their type II diabetes than with medications alone or even with a combination of medications and today's standard dietary advice.

During these years of our own experience with this health challenge, we've been open-minded to well-meaning advisors, but have also tested the results of what we've eaten. We've taken scientific measurements daily to determine the actual results of following their advice. It has only been through taking and making note of these measurements that we've been able to sort out the practical realities from the popular myths. It has been through recognizing and clearly delineating these distinctions that the actual process of the development of type II diabetes has become crystal clear to us. It has only been by coming to this clear understanding of the unique nature of type II diabetes that we've been able to understand how sharply it contrasts with type I. Now that it's so obvious to us, we simply felt an ethical obligation to pass this information on to the people who need it the most – others with type II diabetes trying to reclaim control of their lives with as little medical intervention as possible.

There are some great books on the market that allude to the role of carbohydrate metabolism and diabetes but almost invariably they're aimed at a weight-loss audience. These include the Atkins-type concepts – adequate protein (as opposed to high protein), low carbohydrate, low glycemic index eating approaches. One of the better books on this subject is one called *Protein Power* by Dr. Michael Eades and Dr. Mary Dan Eades. In chapter 3 of the latter, they give an exceptionally good explanation of type II diabetes, better in fact, than in any of the medical texts I've ever read. It's a well-referenced text, presenting ample scientific documentation for even the most discerning of critical thinkers.

This book takes the carbohydrate/protein concept a step farther in its treatment of understanding diabetes, type II especially. It's only by understanding what it is, how it develops, how it progresses, and what is happening with the organs in your body during its development that you'll be able to sift through the advice of writers, nutritionists, radio and TV personalities and even doctors to separate the truth from their unfortunate oversights; oversights that could ultimately cost you your health, if not your limbs or even your life. By the time you finish reading this book, you should understand type II diabetes better than many healthcare professionals and professional nutritionists in the United States. Most importantly, you'll have better control of your own life, secure in the knowledge that you know what's going on in your own body, what to do about it and you won't have to rely on anybody, regardless of their credentials, who does not have a personal reason to understand it as well as you do.

Interestingly enough, dealing effectively with type II diabetes as outlined in this book has several pleasant side effects as well, for instance, weight loss and weight redistribution. Any healthcare professional will agree that there is a close association between excess weight and type II diabetes. But most mistakenly believe that extra weight causes, or contributes to, the diabetes when, in fact, I'm convinced that the extra weight AND the diabetes are BOTH symptoms of the same carbohydrate intolerance, rather than one of these symptoms causing the other. Why is that important? Because losing weight with a low-fat diet (if you can) will probably not achieve the desired results in controlling type II diabetes nearly as well as can be achieved by controlling both the diabetes and the weight with a limited intake of carbohydrates.

People also report feeling not so bloated after meals, sleeping better, reduced snoring, reduction or elimination of nighttime reflux, eliminating cravings, more even energy throughout the day, not being so crabby and depressed, lowered serum cholesterol and lowered blood pressure, to name a few.

In order for you to fully understand this process, you'll need to understand some of the body parts, what their normal jobs are and what happens when things go wrong. So there will be some technical stuff in the coming chapters, but I'll keep it as entertaining as I can while still explaining it in enough detail for you to completely understand the material.

If you're like I am when I read new material, as you read this, it will make a lot of sense to you at the time, but when you try to explain it to somebody later, you might get a little confused. So if you suffer from type II diabetes or somebody in your immediate family does, I urge you to keep at least one copy of this book in your home at all times so you can refer to it when the need arises. I personally think it's also a good idea to keep an extra copy on hand because people will ask you about what you're doing and it will be much easier to lend them a copy of the book than it will be to try to explain the whole thing to them or to lose your personal copy by letting it out of your home. (Lent books have a habit of disappearing permanently, even with the best of the borrowers' intentions.)

I hope that this book will give you the tools you need to stay healthily independent from all the nutritional and diabetic authorities' advice and the fads that go around. I hope it gives you what you need to stay well-grounded in the scientific facts surrounding diabetes, especially type II, and to give you a complete understanding of exactly what it is, how it works and how you can actively minimize its influence on you. I sincerely believe that the truths of the concepts in this book have the potential to "set you free." If the things you've been doing haven't been producing the results you're trying to achieve, then the only obvious course of action is to look for a more effective approach. You may want to try this one. It works amazingly well for Linda, my patients and me. We believe it can work for others as well. Let your own body be the judge!

Contrasting Type I and Type II Diabetes

The first thing that you absolutely have to understand about type II diabetes is that it's very different from type I. Now that may seem overly obvious, but there are a tremendous number of people who are considered medical experts whose understanding of this concept is dangerously incomplete. Consequently, and unfortunately, the information that they give us is erroneous and can actually cause the type II diabetic real and measurable harm, unnecessary suffering and even early death!

To help you understand these important differences, let's start by defining some of the basic things type I and type II diabetes have in common, then, we'll clearly delineate the differences so that you'll have the understanding you'll need to determine for yourself how valid any particular "expert's" opinions and recommendations are.

Both type I and type II diabetics share some common symptoms: polydypsia, polyphasia, and polyuria – meaning constant thirst, constant hunger and a frequent need to urinate, respectively. These symptoms don't just happen at random, on their own. There are specific body processes going on that make these symptoms occur.

Insulin, a substance manufactured and secreted by the pancreas, carries glucose, also known as blood sugar, out of the blood stream and into our cells. In type I diabetes, there's not enough of this insulin being released from the pancreas to carry the blood sugar out of the blood and into the cells where it can be used for energy.

Glucose, or blood sugar, is the only food that our cells use to produce energy. Therefore, when there isn't enough insulin to carry the blood sugar into the cells, the cells are literally starving. When the cells are starving, as in the case of the diabetic, the person naturally experiences constant hunger.

Everything we eat is converted to blood sugar for fuel, constituents for rebuilding our cells, and some waste products. Carbohydrates, fats and proteins are all converted to blood sugar. I want to make a special point here to address the advice of "experts" who proclaim that you need to have a certain amount of carbohydrates in your diet. You don't, because again, everything you eat (except for fiber) is converted into glucose - blood sugar.

All sugars are carbohydrates. All of them, including glucose. In fact, glucose is the most concentrated carbohydrate there is. When you eat meat, it's converted to glucose (plus building blocks and by-products). When you eat fat, it's converted into glucose (and by-products). When you eat carbohydrates, they're simply broken down into a simpler form — glucose (and by-products). So regardless of what you eat, you'll get carbohydrates from it in the end-form of blood sugar – glucose. The only difference in the glucose you get from various foods is how quickly it gets into your blood stream after you eat.

Herein lies the danger for type II diabetics. That is, getting carbohydrates in too great a quantity and in too great a concentration too fast. The only way to prevent this is for you to eat foods that are converted only very slowly into glucose — preferably fats, proteins and very low glycemic index vegetables and fruits. Some type II diabetics may be able to tolerate a few carbohydrates, but getting your glucose from carbohydrate foods is strictly a matter of personal choice and absolutely not a true dietary necessity! This should be great news for people who like creamy foods, bacon with breakfast and thick, juicy steaks.

Type II diabetics experience chronic hunger like type I diabetics, but the bodily processes creating that hunger are quite different. The type II diabetic's pancreas has typically been trained to produce far too much insulin. This creates its own dangers. Too much insulin can cause a condition called, "insulin shock." In the presence of insulin levels that are habitually too high, in order to prevent the occurrence of insulin shock, our body's cells develop a resistance to the insulin as a means of survival. Unfortunately, when the cells become resistant to insulin, they prevent themselves from receiving the vital blood sugar – glucose – as food for converting to energy. The result in this case is also cell starvation and is experienced as hunger and sometimes, pathological, rapid weight loss.

So type II diabetes patients may suffer the same hunger symptoms as the type I diabetic, but the hunger experienced in type I and type II are the result of two very different – actually opposite – causes.

The type I diabetic's hunger is from a lack of insulin. The type II's is from too much insulin and the resulting development of insulin resistance.

These conditions simply cannot be treated the same way by just administering more insulin. While insulin helps the type I diabetic, it only contributes to degeneration in the type II. Therefore, treatment and dietary recommendations that may benefit the type I diabetic patient would actually contribute to worsening the problem in the type II. I cannot over-emphasize the importance of this distinction between the two! Knowing this difference and working with it consciously can make your life far more comfortable, healthy and fun!

In either case, whether there's no insulin to carry the blood sugar into the cells or the cells just won't let the blood sugar in, in addition to hunger, other symptoms develop. One is obviously too much sugar in the blood. Your digestive system does its job to convert your foods to glucose (and by-products) and deposits it into your blood as blood sugar to be carried to all the cells in your body to feed them and provide energy. Too much sugar in the blood actually draws moisture out of the body's tissues, however, like sugar curing or salting a piece of meat to preserve it. When this moisture is drawn out of the body's tissues and held in the blood stream, the result is, predictably, thirst. Your body's tissues lose the vital water necessary to perform the functions of sustaining life and health.

Being thirsty isn't the only concern either. When there is too much moisture being drawn out of your body's tissues, being deposited into your blood stream and stored there, the kidneys have to work overtime to remove all that excess. When all that blood sugar pulls too much moisture from the body's tissues, the kidneys have to work overtime to keep the blood from becoming too diluted. So both type I and type II diabetic patients experience a frequent urge to urinate because, in both cases, the excess blood sugar has the same, moisture robbing, blood-diluting effects, even though the reasons for them occurring are opposite.

These aren't just symptoms to be manipulated with drugs – drugs to lower blood sugar or suppress the appetite; or diuretics, or anti-diuretics – drugs that manipulate your urge to urinate. In the long-run, these drugs only contribute to your problem(s) because they only address isolated symptoms without addressing the underlying processes causing those symptoms.

Type I diabetes is often referred to as Juvenile Onset Diabetes (JOD). Type II is often called Adult Onset Diabetes (AOD) even though type II diabetes is now showing up in younger and younger populations. JOD usually starts in childhood following illness or infection. In JOD, the pancreas has been damaged so badly by the illness that it can't produce adequate amounts of insulin any more. So JOD is a "disease" of insulin deficiency, regardless of the age at which one actually acquires it. It's pretty straight forward and its treatment is obvious – administer insulin.

Type II or AOD, is a very different situation! AOD is the end-result of a series of survival strategies for which the body has become extremely adept. In fact, the body has become so effective at these survival strategies that it over-anticipates what will be happening and over-responds with inappropriate verve. We can think of AOD as the end result of an evolution process that occurs in one individual over a single lifetime.

In ancient days, before the age of commercial processing and easy access to foods, humans ate foods much closer to their natural state. Even in agricultural societies, people ate what came out of the fields with only the barest of preparations. Flour was probably the most processed food they consumed. Even then, until within the past couple of centuries, flour was mostly whole grain rather than refined, bleached, white flour.

The way our foods came to us in centuries and millennia past was in a more balanced state. They had the complete compliment of all their natural components. This is an important concept to comprehend if you want to really understand type II Diabetes. The carbohydrate concentrations in these natural foods were very balanced as contrasted to today's refined and highly altered foods.

When we shop for today's foods from the grocer's shelf, we find that they have far greater concentrations of carbohydrates than the more balanced foods of the past. In earlier centuries, when people wanted something sweet, they reached for a piece of tree-ripened or vine-ripened fruit. Having refined sugar available to add to foods was something of a luxury until about 150 years ago. Many people had it on hand, for sure, but they used it far more sparingly then and they worked it off quickly and efficiently with the strenuous activities required in those times just for daily living. Vegetables typically came from a nearby garden. People usually picked them ripe as well. Today, our vegetables are picked green and ripened during the shipping and display period. Foods in the past were mainly fresh, unprocessed and rich with all the fully developed enzymes and other nutrients these foods should contain in their naturally ripened state.

However, it was difficult for everybody back then to have enough food that way, year round, and in sufficient abundance. At the same time, farmers weren't always able to sell all of their goods before a certain amount would spoil. So there were people missing out on both ends of the spectrum. That, of course, led to developing the modern systems of hybridizing crops to maximize resistance to shipping damage and to increase their shelf life. Food merchants also developed systems to extract only the tastiest parts of foods and to eliminate the rest or use it for other purposes. But in that process, too many foods have lost their natural balance. These imbalances leave us vulnerable to ill health.

For instance, *"Sugar Blues,"* a book that was a best seller in the 1970's, reported that when the British first arrived in India, they weren't at all pleased with having to eat brown rice. They thought it was too crude and unsophisticated. They only wanted to eat the processed, polished, white rice. They left the brown rice for the servants. After a time, pellagra and pernicious anemia began to show up in the English there in India, but the Indian servants had no such problems. It perplexed the doctors of their day to no end. After extensive investigation, they discovered that the refining / polishing process was removing not only the unsightly brown covering on the rice, it was also removing vital B vitamins. The British were eating plenty of rice, but an unbalanced form of it, not the whole grain. They were getting their bellies full and satisfying their immediate hunger, but they were starving certain body systems because of the imbalance of their main food source.

In 20th and 21st century America, our food has been processed far beyond anything our ancestors could possibly have imagined! Most of this food processing has to do with taste appeal and shelf life, but with little or no intent toward offering its greatest nutritional value. There are two primary ways to process food that enhance both its taste and increase its shelf life – using salt and using sugar. Any commercial food supplier knows this very well.

Salt fell into unearned disrepute many years ago, however, due to assumptions of negative effects on blood volume, blood pressure, and a perceived potential for contributing to strokes, sparking the "low-sodium" labeling craze. Today, however, salty foods are still huge sellers in America.

Sugar, the other tasty preservative, and the more popular of the two, is by far the most commonly added ingredient in commercial foods, across the board! Evidence suggests that because of its omnipresence in our foods, it's the initiating culprit in the development of AOD.

To understand how AOD develops, let's look at the relationship of sugar, simple carbohydrates, complex carbohydrates and blood sugar. Blood sugar, also called glucose, is a single-molecule, a simple sugar, the simplest form of sugar in the body. Absolutely everything that we ever eat, except fiber, is converted to glucose in our digestive system. Sugar(s), including table sugar, mannose, dextrose, mannitol, xylitol, dextrin, maltodextrin, fructose, (and other ingredients ending in "ol," "rin" or "ose" which are included in this category) are very simple, small, basic, sugar molecules. They break down into their component parts in the digestive tract, including their glucose component, in as little as 30 minutes.

I'm going to assign you some homework so you can fully grasp the importance of this last paragraph. Lots of people believe that they're restricting the sugar or the carbohydrates they eat because they don't see the word "sugar" on a label. Walk down any aisle in the grocery store, pick up any package or jar of food and read the label. Look for "sugar" then look for corn syrup and all ingredients ending with 'rin, 'ose, and 'ol. You'll probably be shocked to discover how much sugar you actually do consume on a daily basis, sugars labeled by unfamiliar names perhaps, but sugars nonetheless.

Next, go to the desserts aisles. Look at some pastries, cakes, pies, jellies, jams, and all sorts of sweet dessert foods. Look at the carbohydrate count per serving. Look at several different items so you get a feel for the average amounts of carbs in these highly sugared foods.

Then go down the aisles and pick up packaged dinner foods like pastas and pasta sauces, breads, mixes of all sorts, gravies and pre-packaged dinners. Look at the carbohydrate count on these foods. Look at the "rin's," "ol's," "ose's" and corn syrup in these foods too. You'll be amazed to find how high these foods are in both overall carbohydrates and sugars by other names. They often contain nearly as many carbohydrates as the sweet desserts you looked at earlier. With carbohydrate comparisons being so close, it's like eating sweet desserts with every meal we eat! Is it any wonder then that our carbohydrate metabolism becomes overwhelmed?

Simple carbohydrates are molecules that break down into sugars, including glucose, very quickly. Again, these simple carbohydrates are typically converted into glucose within 30 minutes to two hours. Non-sugar, simple carbohydrates are just one step more complicated than sugars themselves. We find simple carbohydrates in all fruits, grains like corn, rice and wheat and in starchy or sweet vegetables - potatoes, sweet potatoes, tomatoes, carrots and peas, and in breads – some of the most prevalent staples of the American diet.

As carbohydrate molecules become larger and more complicated, they enter the category of foods that have "complex carbohydrates." Because these are larger molecular structures and more complex, it requires a little more effort and takes the digestive system a little longer to break them down into simple sugars and glucose – blood sugar. These carbohydrates typically take about two hours to break down and their glucose is released into the blood stream a bit more gradually over those two hours instead of just 30 minutes like the simpler sugars. Whole grains and pastas are said to be in this "complex carbohydrates" category. So glucose is the simplest sugar - blood sugar. Simple sugars break down into glucose quickly. They take about 30 minutes. Complex carbohydrates take about 2 hours to break down into glucose. The more complicated the molecule, the longer it takes to convert into glucose.

Now that you have a basic understanding of the scale of simplicity and complexity of carbohydrates ranging from the complex carbs in pastas and grains down to simple sugars by any name, and glucose – simple blood sugar, let's look at how they all contribute to type II diabetes, AOD.

One more time, all food is converted to glucose. Glucose is the food that feeds every cell in the entire human body. Whether we're eating pie (carbohydrates), butter (fat) or a juicy steak (protein), it will all eventually become glucose (plus some "building blocks" and waste products). Glucose is the food that the cells use to produce energy.

When we eat, and our food is digested, then converted to glucose, the presence of that glucose in the blood ("blood sugar") triggers the pancreas to produce insulin and introduce it into our blood stream. Why? Because insulin is what carries glucose out of our blood streams and into our bodies' cells. Without insulin, glucose has a very hard time finding its way into our cells. Strenuous exercise is about the only way we can force it in without the insulin. It's only logical then that glucose (blood sugar) would trigger the release of insulin. It's our bodies' method for feeding itself.

Blood sugar not only feeds the cells, it has other effects in the body too. If the blood sugar level is too high, water is pulled out of the body's tissues as you read earlier. That causes profound thirst. At the same time, the kidneys have to work overtime to get rid of the extra water in the blood. So the person has to urinate a lot. Our bodies innately know this.

On the other hand, if blood sugar levels are too low, we experience hunger and eventually all of the symptoms that accompany hypoglycemia (low blood sugar) — nervousness, hypothermia (feeling cold), headaches, confusion, pronounced irritability and at the extreme, convulsions and coma.

To keep our blood sugar levels in this narrow range that's safe for the body, insulin has to be released in amounts that match the glucose that's expected to come flooding into the blood stream after we eat, but not so much as to cause it to plummet too low.

Let's go back to the grocery store items again. In ancient times, when foods weren't processed, the carbohydrate content was mostly the complex type of carbohydrates. Simple sugars were a rarity, a luxury. Our bodies were accustomed to little or no sugar and the carbohydrates we did consume were mostly complex ones that entered our systems as glucose slowly and gradually.

Not today! We find high concentrations of sugars and simple carbohydrates in the majority of all packaged foods now. In fact, if they don't have sugars or salt in them, they simply can't compete in a market that evaluates everything in terms of pleasant taste to the exclusion of any real nutritional value. These high concentrations of carbohydrates and sugars digest almost instantly and pour massive amounts of glucose into the blood all at once. This has become the rule rather than the exception. Remember, in the blood, glucose is blood sugar.

Since high concentrations of blood sugar are as dangerous as abnormally low amounts of blood sugar, and because today's American diet contains such inordinately high amounts of carbohydrates and sugars, it's vital for the pancreas to recognize the presence of carbohydrates immediately in order to anticipate the high concentrations that are coming with today's typical meal or snack. The pancreas trains itself well over time and becomes extremely good at this, especially in those people who develop AOD. Recognizing that when the person eats nearly anything, there will be large concentrations of carbohydrates coming, and very quickly, the pancreas begins to condition itself to release massive amounts of insulin at the slightest hint of carbohydrates to prevent dangerously high blood sugar levels and the damage they can create.

But the pancreas gets so proficient at this that it starts to over-anticipate. Not only does it secrete enough insulin to bring the blood sugar level down to normal, the huge amounts of insulin released actually cause the blood sugar to plummet past a safe level and even farther down into an abnormally low blood sugar condition (hypoglycemia). If the blood sugar drops low enough, the person can lose consciousness. It's not a good thing at all!

One of the symptoms of low blood sugar is hunger as we explained earlier. Insulin also delivers blood sugar to the hypothalamus. That's the part of your brain that registers hunger and being full or satisfied. When excess insulin has removed too much blood sugar from the blood making it unavailable to the hypothalamus, the brain registers it as hunger. Then, because of the hunger, we unwittingly crave more foods and snacks, usually carbohydrate-rich ones. And the cycle repeats over and over.

So when someone's pancreas has become overly responsive with its insulin release, the result is usually constant hunger. People in this situation will eat until they're full and, within a half an hour or so, find themselves hanging on the refrigerator door, hungry again, even though they're still full, not knowing why. They'll have days when they're not all that hungry until they eat something in the morning. Then all day long they're munching on something, but never getting satisfied. They go to bed stuffed, but still hungry. This is a classic sign of a person who is hyperinsulinemic, pre-diabetic — whose pancreas habitually releases far too much insulin and whose cells have become resistant to that insulin.

In these people, instead of releasing adequate amounts of insulin to manage the blood sugar slowly and efficiently, the pancreas is mostly either all the way on or all the way off. The presence of blood sugar simply turns it on and it pumps insulin out in inappropriately massive doses, which in turn, causes the blood sugar to plummet past normal, safe levels and the cells to become more and more resistant to insulin. Then more insulin is need to overcome the resistance and the cells become even more resistant - and the cycle spirals out of control.

Ironically, if these people had fasting glucose tests done in a medical laboratory, they would likely read normal; however, if they looked at the insulin levels, the insulin would be very high. Unfortunately, very few doctors ever think to order tests for insulin levels.

In this pre-diabetic person with hyperinsulinemia (hypoglycemia), or type II diabetic steadily gaining weight, the insulin is actually carrying most of this blood sugar into the cells despite their resistance. However, any time there's more glucose coming into the cells than the cells are actually using, the body turns it into fat and stores it. Even though there are certainly adequate amounts of food coming into their bodies, the type II diabetic or pre-diabetic can always be hungry. And even in the presence of this insatiable hunger, the body is storing food, in the form of fat, to be used at a future date when and if the need should arise. I believe that this is the number one cause of obesity in both humans and our pets today. If we want to fatten beef or pork, do we feed them protein or fat? No! We feed them corn – a very high-*carbohydrate* food!

Understand that there is a known relationship between excess weight and type II diabetes. BUT! I'm convinced that it's not a causative relationship! In other words, people with AOD are typically overweight, but the excess weight is a *symptom* of the diabetes rather than the *cause* of the diabetes! Conversely, experts tell us that if an AOD patient loses weight, the diabetes will improve. The improvement of the diabetes isn't because they lost weight, however. It's because the most effective way that a type II diabetic can actually lose weight is to change what's happening in the hunger, blood-sugar, insulin loop by limiting their intake of carbohydrates, either purposely or incidentally. The excess weight of type II diabetics is just as much of a symptom of the process we're describing as is the diabetes itself. Clearly stated – the weight does not cause the diabetes. The process that becomes AOD causes the excess weight!

Our bodies are innately very wise. They recognize the problems of always being hungry, feeding ourselves and storing all of this extra fat that can kill us! So our bodies do something very smart to control all of that excess, unused fat being stored in our cells. The cells start to develop a resistance to the insulin! What does this accomplish? It prevents the blood sugar from being carried out of the blood and into the cells, especially since the cells are already full, or even over-full. This insulin resistance is a survival technique meant to prevent us from getting so massively fat that we choke to death!

Let's recap everything up to here. Excess carbohydrates and sugars are everywhere in our modern, American diets. Constant, habitual consumption of these high concentrations of carbohydrates train the pancreas to pump out huge amounts of insulin in response.

The huge amounts of insulin make us fat and, simultaneously, keep us hungry all the time. In order to survive this downward spiraling process, our cells become resistant to insulin. Now what?

If the blood sugar can't get into the cells, we'll stay hungry and probably eat a lot ("polyphasia"), but the blood sugar doesn't go into the cells, it stays in the blood. This high blood sugar concentration dries out our tissues and causes constant thirst ("polydypsia") and pulls water into the blood stream. The excess water in the blood stream needs to be filtered out and excreted in the urine ("polyuria") so that the blood doesn't become too diluted. At this point the kidneys will work like crazy to try to keep the blood at the right consistency. In fact, it will become so proficient at pulling the excess water out of the blood at the slightest signal to do so that it will even learn to identify what's making it attract so much water – excess blood sugar! Then our well-trained kidneys will even begin to pass the blood sugar out in the urine too. *Sugar in the urine is the number one hallmark of diabetes – type I or type II.*

Now for a little test. Knowing what you now know about how type II develops, what would you say to a person who tells you that a type II diabetic needs to have five servings of carbohydrates per day (as recommended in the standard Food Pyramid)? Will that help the type II diabetic or contribute to the problem? Answer: IT WILL CAUSE MORE HARM! It can be no other way, regardless of the good intentions or the credentials of people who think you should have a "balanced diet," using the nationally accepted Food Pyramid as their model. Carbohydrates are poison for the type II diabetic! Again I want to reiterate that eating carbohydrate foods specifically is not necessary because everything we eat is converted to glucose, the most concentrated carbohydrate there is.

What's the role of fats in the diet for type II diabetics? Let me illustrate with a question. If you were going to fly to another state, would you want a trained pilot that was an experienced flyer or a brand new, student pilot? If you were going to build a new house, would you want an experienced builder to do it or would you prefer a new apprentice carpenter who had never built anything? The answer, of course, is obvious. What's that have to do with fats and diabetics?

I refer again to the "experts" who make the connection between excess weight and diabetics. They assume that consuming fat is the cause of gaining the weight and that reducing fats in your diet, therefore, can help you lose weight to control the diabetes! That would be logical if it were true. But I've just explained that the weight gain of diabetics is primarily from carbohydrate consumption and that the fat they store is part of the problem rather than the cause.

I've also explained that all foods we eat, except fiber, become glucose. The fat that we store is actually meant to become glucose later on – when we need it. But as long as we're consuming carbohydrates and spinning the cycle of carbs, insulin and diabetes, there's absolutely no need for the body to use fat *because it's still in the process of making it*!

So what's the solution? We can use the trainability of the body to our advantage. Let's go at it from two very distinct approaches: First, stop contributing to the proliferation of fat by discontinuing it's source – sugars and other carbohydrates – as much as you possibly can. Will you be able to eliminate them altogether? I don't think that that's even possible in America unless all you ever eat is meat and that wouldn't be advisable. But start by getting your daily carbohydrate intake to 30 grams or less. That includes sauces, condiments, dressings, snacks, drinks – everything. Your body's cells will soon recognize that they don't have excess blood sugar to turn into fat. In fact, your blood sugar will level out over the day and stay in a more normal range because those simple molecules of the sugars and carbohydrates will not be available to spike your insulin levels any more. Your body will have to begin to depend on the other two food sources for its glucose – fats and proteins.

Fats are very complicated molecules compared to the simplicity of carbohydrates, and proteins are even more complex than fats. The result is that when your body uses either fat or protein as its glucose source, the glucose is fed to the blood stream, not in massive, concentrated doses, but slowly, over time, in small quantities.

If we want to kill lots of birds with a single stone, training our bodies to use fats as its source of glucose is an effective way to do it. Can we train our bodies to use fat as its food source by eating carbohydrates? Absolutely not. That *makes* fat! Can we train our bodies to use fat as its food source by restricting our fats? Can you train an Olympic runner for successful competition by having him sit on a couch all day? In order to train our bodies to use fats as their food source, we must specifically give them fats while we dramatically restrict carbohydrates! In the absence of simple molecules to break down into glucose (carbohydrates) our bodies resort to the next most available source – fat. By including fats in our diet, we train our bodies to rely on fat (including its own) as a food source. And because fats break down more slowly, we don't have resulting spikes of insulin response and subsequent over-lowering of the blood sugar causing us constant hunger. Our energy level smoothes out over the day, we're far less hungry and hungry far less often. We can eat less and actually be more satisfied!

If you're a type II diabetic, it's vital to include fats in your diet if you want to train it to use fats instead of relying on carbohydrates and to decrease your weight.

But there's a balance you must observe here too. Fat has 9 calories per gram compared to only 4 calories per gram of carbohydrates. If we want to reduce our weight, we can't use this recommendation about including fats in our diets as carte blanche to indulge so deeply in fat consumption that we're getting all of our glucose from what we eat and not requiring our bodies to mobilize some of their own fat stores. The amount of fats we can eat without gaining weight varies for different people, but it's usually a fairly generous amount.

You'll want to eat enough fats to train your body to use them as a food source instead of relying on carbs, but you don't want to be consuming so many fats that your body stores them as temporarily unusable fat in your cells.

The best way to discover what this amount is for you personally is to purchase some "Ketostix" from your local drug store. They measure ketones in your urine. Ketones are a by-product of burning fat. Use the Ketostix to measure the ketones in your urine on a daily basis, preferably at, or near, the same time daily.

Very high concentrations of ketones can be a sign of danger. This isn't necessarily because of the ketones themselves, but because of the processes that those high concentrations indicate. That being said, our goal is to give ourselves tangible, measurable evidence that our bodies are using fat as a glucose source by monitoring the amount of ketones in the urine. If the body isn't producing any ketones at all in the urine, you can bet that the body is using very little or no fat at all as fuel. On the other hand, in order to err on the safe side, we don't want our ketones to be so high that there could be potential problems.

With your Ketostix, pick a time of day to take your measurements. I do it in the evenings at my first urination after I get home or around 6 - 8 PM. Morning urine is concentrated as the body has been working in a very different mode all night, so I personally believe that the evening reading is the most useful and accurate.

When you read the stick (determining the color) it should ideally read in the "moderate" range. This will show that you are definitely using fats as a fuel, whether that fat is dietary fat or fat from your own body. If you want to use the Ketostix to determine if you are burning your body's own fat, it requires a little more personal attention to your readings. You must experiment with your diet (what you eat on a daily basis) and note the readings every day. Keep close track of what you eat during the day and what the corresponding reading is that evening. Weigh yourself after you've showered (or bathed) and gone to the bathroom every morning to see if you are losing, gaining, or maintaining your weight. After a time, you'll recognize that once your carbohydrate intake surpasses a certain amount during the course of a day, a pattern of "trace" or "zero" ketones will develop, and you nearly always stop losing weight, or even gain again. Simply reduce your carbohydrate intake to achieve the ketone readings that correspond to previous readings when you have actually been losing weight.

Once you've determined the carbohydrate amount your body can handle before you stop losing weight, you can experiment with the amount of fat you consume as well. To find the amount of fat your body can handle before it starts becoming extra body weight, be very strict about your carbohydrate intake to keep it in the "losing weight" range on your Ketostix for several days. Then vary your fat intake for several days and monitor the results with your scales. When your fat intake causes you to gain weight (if you can even consume that much fat in a day), you have determined what your personal cut-off point is. This valuable tool is great for helping you to have individualized, personal feedback for what works for you and what doesn't, what levels your body can handle and what is simply beyond your body's ability to use.

Incidentally, when type II diabetics adhere to a diet of restricted carbohydrates, moderate fat and adequate protein, as you will see in later chapters, cholesterol levels often normalize, blood pressure often settles to a more ideal number and weight loss is merely a wonderfully welcome side effect!

Cholesterol, Facts and Fiction

Unfortunately, there's a lot of dangerous misinformation about cholesterol floating around in both the professional healthcare community and the general public. It's in the magazines and the newspapers. It's on TV and the internet. It's even in doctors' offices. You see article after article in one medium after another, each quoting the other, perpetuating these unfortunate and dangerous misunderstandings without validation. Just a little education in biochemistry tells us that something just isn't adding up. When I started doing my research for this book, I was amazed at how simple the truth about this subject really is and how well it's actually backed up by quality medical research and good-old-fashioned, common sense.

For instance, award-winning author, Sheldon Zerden, lists more than 100 misunderstandings held out to be facts by many, if not the majority, of healthcare professionals today, in his book *"The Cholesterol Hoax."* I was particularly impressed by this particular work because every incorrect concept he addresses, he refutes with a referenced study. I highly recommend this as required reading material for anyone who is concerned about cholesterol levels.

I was also appalled to discover how completely this basic, scientific information about cholesterol is ignored by the very people who should be the most reliable experts – healthcare professionals.

In this chapter, you'll read some myth-busting, scientific information about cholesterol that's based on proven facts instead of unsubstantiated opinions. You'll see information that's vital for every person to know who's interested in his or her overall health – information that's not based merely on insurance charts or drug company sales strategies.

The first thing you'll need to know about cholesterol is what it's *not*. It's not a death agent that you need to eliminate from your body as much as possible -- not by any stretch of the imagination! In fact, without adequate amounts of cholesterol, you would die very quickly. Your body builds your hormones with cholesterol – all three types of estrogen, testosterone and progesterone, just to name a few.

Your body makes bile acids with cholesterol, a substance manufactured in the liver to help enable you to digest fatty foods.

Cholesterol is the initial precursor for building neurotransmitters, the chemicals that enable one nerve cell to send its messages to the next. Your entire brain is a giant bundle of interacting nerve cells. So cholesterol is critical for healthy brain and nerve function. It's said that 80 percent of the brain is cholesterol! (Which should give you some insight into the very real dangers of artificially lowering your cholesterol with drugs like Lipitor, Zocor and other cholesterol lowering drugs!) This is why so many people experience mental fogginess when using anti-cholesterol drugs and are surprised at the sudden clarity of mental functions when they discontinue taking them.

E. C. had been a chiropractic patient of mine for some time. Always wanting to take the best care of his health that he can, he didn't hesitate when his medical doctor put him on a statin, a cholesterol lowering medication. During the months that followed, at his regular chiropractic appointments, he complained of mental distortion and confusion that was progressively getting worse.

Frustrated, he did some research on his own to find out if the anti-cholesterol drugs might be involved. In the process, he discovered references to the impaired brain function/statin connection. He immediately decided to discontinue the medication. Within days of quitting, he told me that his mental function had become "amazingly clearer" and he has reported no lack of mental clarity for more than two years now.

Cholesterol is what gives skin its ability to shed water. It's the precursor (building material) for your body to make vitamin D, an essential component for healthy bone density and for fighting osteoporosis. It's a key element for your body to be able to grow and to repair itself. Every cell in your body needs cholesterol to perform its normal functions and to reproduce new cells.

Cholesterol is obviously NOT the villain that so many portray it to be!

If your cholesterol level is too low, you actually increase your risk of death from health conditions other than heart disease, conditions like strokes or cancer. In fact, falling cholesterol levels are a distinct marker for cancer! It may be true that the lower your cholesterol levels are, the lower your risk of heart attack, but once it falls below a certain point (a number that may shock you), you run an increased risk of death from other causes, such as stroke and cancer.

In Sheldon Verdon's book, he refers to *The Lancet,* 1974, 1, 523 Rose, G., et. al. stating that "31 studies including Framington, 7 countries studies and the giant multiple risk factor intervention trial (MRFIT) reported higher cancer or total death rates with subjects who have lower cholesterol levels. ... The majority of studies lean toward a negative correlation, suggesting that low cholesterol levels may facilitate the growth of cancers or other diseases."

So what's the ideal level of cholesterol? Drs. Michael and Mary Dan Eades suggest it's about 190 and that the ideal and safest range is actually between 180 and 200. According to this paradigm, your risk of death from too little cholesterol is actually about the same at 140 as it is from too much cholesterol at 240! So despite the urgings of doctors and the drug manufacturers to reduce your cholesterol to very low levels, lowering it below 180 is a foolhardy and dangerous thing to do! For every number increment you lower your serum cholesterol below 180, it adds as much risk to your life as raising it an increment above 200. Your heart is certainly important for staying alive, true, but it's only one of many essential body organs we have to consider that are also required for maintaining life!

"Good" Cholesterol and "Bad" cholesterol:

Although there are other forms of cholesterol, the two that we're most concerned with in this discussion are low density lipoproteins (LDLs) and high density lipoproteins (HDLs). The LDLs are considered the "bad" ones. The HDLs are considered the "good' ones. But healthy concentrations of cholesterol involve more than mere counts. Ratios are just as important, if not more so.

When we go to the doctor's office or the lab to have blood work done so that we can see what our cholesterol levels might be, we have to look at the total cholesterol number, the HDL number and the LDL number. Then we need to do a little math. Divide your total cholesterol count by your HDL count. Ideally, the number should be 4 or less. Next divide your LDL count by your HDL count. The ideal number should be 3 or less for maximum health. Write these ratios down so that you can remember them and keep an on-going record of them. Many report cholesterol levels becoming more ideal, without drugs, when they follow the dietary suggestions in this book.

J. For instance, discovered on her initial work-up at her doctor's office that her cholesterol was well over 700, certainly high by anyone's standard. The doctor put her on a special diet specifically designed to lower cholesterol and he prescribed two cholesterol-lowering medications. Although the strategy did lower it, it was certainly inadequate. It only brought it down to the upper 400's.

She decided to go to another doctor. Further testing showed that in addition to the high cholesterol, she also had an elevated blood sugar level. Her new doctor took her off of all of her cholesterol-lowering medications and recommended a diet similar to the one suggested in this book - very low carbohydrate with adequate protein and fat. Her next appointment showed that her cholesterol level had dropped to just under 190 and her blood sugar to under 100! Cases like this are common.

Lets look at another, though hypothetical, scenario that happens all too often when people are concerned about cholesterol and diet and keeping their cholesterol under control. A man goes to the doctor who discovers from his blood tests that his total cholesterol level is at 240. (HDL 60 and LDL 180) The doctor, seeing that this level is undesirably high, recommends a specific type of diet and says that it's guaranteed to get cholesterol down to 200 if he follows it to the letter. This patient is concerned and wants to do the right thing, so he follows the diet very closely and sure enough, when he re-tests his blood for cholesterol levels, the new reading is all the way down to 200 (HDL 45 and LDL 155). That's certainly a much better total number, according to the general charts, but is it all good? Let's look a little closer.

If this patient's HDL was at 60 on his first test result, that would make the ratio 4 (total cholesterol [240] divided by HDL [60] = 4). That's in the ideal range. On the second test, however, the HDL was 45. Even though the total cholesterol count was down, even to an ideal range for a total, the new ratio would have changed to 4.4 (200 total cholesterol divided by 45 HDL = 4.4). The new ratio is actually worse for this patient's health and is leading him toward a more serious risk of heart attack! This isn't good at all. The reason he went to the doctor was because he wanted to lower his cholesterol in the first place — to lower his health risks! So you can plainly see from this example that it's not as simple as just randomly decreasing numbers like the doctors, insurance companies and pharmaceutical salesmen would like for us to believe! Ratios are actually a greater concern than total numbers. There are more bits of information about cholesterol and diet that seem to be myths as well.

An interesting study that was published in *"the Journal of Clinical Endocrinology & Metabolism"* shattered some widely held, current beliefs: There were two groups of people in this particular experiment. They fed one group a high fat, "low carbohydrate" diet (175 grams of carbs per day – a level of carbohydrates still high enough that the majority of diabetics would not be able to handle it on a regular basis without medications). The other group was fed a diet that was low in fat but was high in complex carbohydrates, (the diet currently recommended by most dietitians and healthcare professionals) for two weeks. After the first two weeks, the groups switched diets for the next two weeks. The results were shocking! After two weeks on the high carb, low fat diet, the average total cholesterol was 159 (in the dangerously low range) and the ratio of HDL to LDL (which needs to be 3 or less) was 3.47, a high number.

The group on the high fat, "low carbohydrate" diet had an average cholesterol level of 191 (only one point above the ideal reading) with a ratio of HDL to LDL of 3.31 (still high but much better than the low fat group)!

If the "low carb" diet in this experiment had been limited to 30 grams or less per day, the resulting differences would have probably been far more dramatic.

Healthcare professionals have been admonishing people for years to avoid eggs as if they were pure poison, especially egg yolks, because they contain such high levels of cholesterol. But the prestigious *"New England Journal of Medicine"* published a case study of an 88 year old man who ate an average of twenty five eggs each and every day for thirty years. The medical experts who caution against eating anything containing cholesterol would have expected this man to have had astronomically high levels of cholesterol with a diet like this, but he didn't. His cholesterol levels had remained at an average of 200 for the entire time (he'd been in a nursing home where it was closely monitored for all those years). His HDL to LDL ratio was 3.16 — close to ideal, especially for an 88 year old man! How did he accomplish this amazing feat? How was that even possible? Read on!

In study after study, people have eaten high amounts of fats but their cholesterol levels have stayed unchanged or nearly unchanged. In some of these experiments, subjects have eaten large amounts of cholesterol itself with no change to their cholesterol levels at all. But other studies showed an immediate increase in cholesterol levels with high fat diets and/or high cholesterol intake. So what is it that makes the difference? The answer to that question is so simple, so natural, so healthy and so easy to do that it actually makes some people angry when they discover what it is!

A proven, effective, drug-free, dietary procedure for normalizing cholesterol levels and attaining optimal HDL to LDL levels can be completely summarized in just two simple words: Restrict carbohydrates!

It's certainly safer than any of the prescription cholesterol drugs which can, themselves, cause a host of problems including rheumatoid arthritis-like symptoms and muscle weakness to the point of weakness in the diaphragm and/or weak heart beats – low blood pressure. The onset of symptoms from these cholesterol lowering drugs can appear within hours! In my own practice, I've seen two patients nearly die from the side effects of statin drugs (cholesterol lowering medications) that their regular doctors prescribed for them.

D. E.'s doctor placed him on cholesterol lowering drugs in 1999. Within days, he developed shortness of breath, weakness, abnormally low blood pressure and such severe joint pains throughout his entire body, that he and his wife truly believed he had suddenly developed rheumatoid arthritis overnight! (Which just doesn't happen.)

When we explained rheumatoid arthritis to him, and he understood that it would be rare indeed for it to develop so severely in such a short time, he questioned his druggist about the cholesterol medication. The druggist dismissed the possibility, even though it's a clearly stated side effect in the literature that comes with the drug.

His blood pressure dropped so low that he had difficulty standing. His muscles became so weak that he had difficulty breathing. But his regular doctor agreed with the druggist.

Frightened and losing faith in his doctor, he sought a second opinion with his doctor at the Veteran's Administration hospital. This doctor correctly identified his new problem as side effects of the cholesterol drug and recommended that he discontinue its use. Once he did, the symptoms began to clear up immediately.

We must logically assume, therefore, that a nutritional approach to normalizing cholesterol levels and cholesterol ratios certainly must be a more reasonable and safe approach than using dangerous, cholesterol lowering, prescription drugs and in at least some cases it's possibly even more effective.

How does a low-carbohydrate dietary approach accomplish these very desirable results? Let me explain. When we eat carbohydrates, because they're such simple, easy-to-break-down molecules, they're rapidly converted into their simplest form – glucose – blood sugar – when digested. The presence of blood sugar triggers the release of insulin from the pancreas into the blood stream. The purpose of this insulin is to carry the blood sugar out of the blood stream and into the cells where it's then converted to energy. Carrying the blood sugar out of the blood stream and into the cells, therefore, lowers the blood sugar to achieve normal levels and feeds the cells themselves.

In the United States especially, because our bodies are so adept at dealing with very high amounts and concentrations of carbohydrates in the average diet that many people, especially those who carry extra weight, not only release insulin, they release abnormally high amounts – in fact, massive amounts! This causes some of the most challenging problems in America today including run-away obesity in the public, constant, insatiable hunger and eventual type II diabetes, a major epidemic in this country. Childhood obesity in our society is in epidemic proportions now and I absolutely believe that this is the primary cause.

The presence of insulin in our blood stream also causes the cells in our bodies to produce their own cholesterol inside of themselves, a process described in physiology books as the "cholesterol synthesis pathway." When this happens, the cells ignore any cholesterol that may be present in the blood because they already have enough to perform all their functions. Consequently, the cholesterol remains in the blood ("high serum cholesterol"). This serum cholesterol can in turn cause problems in the heart and the arteries when it combines with homocysteine and in the absence of enough vitamin C and bioflavonoids. You'll read about what are sufficient amounts of vitamin C later in this text.

Researchers, such as Kilmer S. McCully, M. D., author *of "The Homocysteine Revolution,"* determined in the late twentieth century that cholesterol in the arteries is not nearly the culprit it is reputed to be, but rather homocysteine. It appears to be the substance that triggers cholesterol to form plaques in the arteries. Health care professionals who are current in their research of the scientific literature have known this for a number of years. You can buy "homocysteine regulators" (Vitamins B6, B12, Folic acid and Betain) inexpensively at your local health food store.

High levels of insulin also cause an abundance of LDL cholesterol (the "bad" ones).

On the other hand, when we restrict our intake of carbohydrates, decreasing the corresponding insulin response, the cells actually decrease their production of their own cholesterol too and instead, take it out of the blood, lowering serum cholesterol levels.

Low levels of insulin also result in higher levels of HDLs (the "good" ones).

What does all this mean? It means that we've been misled for decades, even if altogether unintentionally, with completely erroneous misinformation about diet and cholesterol. This misleading information has unfortunately been based on assumptions about limited and incomplete observations, rather than on scientifically proven human physiology! It's like the assumption that, "The sun orbits the earth," was an errant conclusion based on limited and incomplete observations. They only had some of the available facts and based their conclusions on that partial information.

What are the scientifically proven facts?

1) High cholesterol levels are NOT the result of eating high cholesterol foods, except when they're eaten in combination with high levels of carbohydrates.

2) We do NOT have to restrict our fat intake to lower our cholesterol levels unless the fat is eaten in combination with high levels of carbohydrates (French fries or doughnuts are prime American examples).

3) Getting our cholesterol levels as low as we possibly can is certainly NOT a desirable or even a healthy thing to do! It's actually a very foolish and dangerous idea! The goal is to achieve IDEAL levels and to have those levels in ideal ratios.

4) The perfect cholesterol level is NOT 160 or 140. It's 190! The safest range is 180 to 200. For every point we reduce the cholesterol reading below 180, we encounter as much additional risk to our health and to our lives as we would by increasing it by a corresponding point above 200. A reading of 140 is as dangerous as 240.

    In the book, *"The Cholesterol Hoax,"* Sheldon Zerden actually quotes several studies suggesting that even these levels are artificially low and undesirable.

5) We can't control our blood sugar levels nor our insulin levels by restricting our intake of FAT! Controlling blood sugar levels can only be done by controlling our intake of carbohydrates. The extra weight is not the *cause* of the carbohydrate intolerance. Excess weight is the *result* of carbohydrate intolerance just like type II diabetes.

6) Complex carbohydrates (pasta, grains, etc.) are not "good" carbohydrates (for type II diabetics) as we're told. They turn to blood sugar too. It just takes an extra hour or two for them to do so. The result is still massively high insulin level responses, producing high cholesterol levels, just like eating sugar.

Then how much do you need to restrict your carbohydrate levels if you want to have ideal cholesterol levels and ideal HDL to LDL ratios?

It will vary from person to person, depending on your individual carbohydrate metabolism. But here are a few guidelines that I suggest.

1) If your personal cholesterol picture is outside of the ideal parameters you've seen here and you want to correct it as quickly as possible, I recommend restricting your carbohydrate intake to 30 grams or less per day for at least three weeks, testing your urine daily in the afternoons or the evenings with "Ketostix" or "Keto-Diastix" (from any drug store) to make sure you're producing at least a small amount of ketones daily and spilling zero amounts of sugar into your urine. Do adjust your carbohydrate intake to keep the ketones below 80 mg/dl, however.

2) After three weeks, add small amounts of carbohydrates each day until you test negative for ketones ("zero"). Then back off on the carbs again, just a little, so that you stay at a level where you test between "trace" and "moderate" on your Ketostix daily. This is where you should stay until you reach your ideal cholesterol profile — 180 to 200 total (190 is ideal). When you have your cholesterol checked, look at all three of the readings: total cholesterol, HDL and LDL. Your LDL divided by HDL should be 3 or less; total cholesterol divided by HDL should be 4 or less.

3) Your fat intake will be of little consequence. In fact, cream or half and half will be better for you than skim milk or 2% because the higher the cream content, the fewer carbohydrates it contains per ounce. Most people have difficulty consuming more fat than is safe because the body reaches a satiety point quickly with fat consumption and you just stop before you get more than is safe (as long as it's NOT being combined with carbohydrates).

4) Enjoy your bacon and eggs or steak and eggs for breakfast but pass on the toast and juice. This is just the opposite of what you've

always been trained to think, right? Our fellow in the nursing home who ate 25 eggs a day ate very little of anything else! There were little or no carbohydrates consumed with his 25 eggs every day. So that's how his cholesterol levels remained nearly perfect despite consuming so much of such a high-cholesterol food!

5) Have all the fatty, juicy steaks you want but pass on the baked potatoes.

6) Have thick, rich, creamy Ranch dressing or vinegar and oil on your salad, but pass on the croutons and the diet raspberry dressing.

7) Take some time to learn the carbohydrate content of all the foods that you would normally include in your daily menus. I've included an abbreviated carbohydrate chart in the back of this book; however, please pick up a more complete Carbohydrate Counter book of some kind at your local book store and take some time to study it well so that you can make good selections at the spur of the moment when you're eating out. You may even want to make flash cards to carry with you for a few months until you really know your foods well without having to look them up.

8) Have a great, thick, juicy hamburger, or even a double, with cheese, but take off the bun and pass on the fries! For instance, according to Burger King's dietary statistics, a Burger King Double Whopper with cheese has 54 grams of carbs with the bun but only 4 grams without the bun!

Oh yes! By the way, you can lose weight this way too! By restricting our carbohydrate intake to 20-30 grams of carbohydrates a day, my wife and I can drop an average of about 1 to 2 pounds a week. It was even more in the beginning. This principle is the driving force behind the Atkins diet, the Protein Power diet and other low-carbohydrate approaches to weight loss. Other popular diets often work because their recommendations include mostly low carbohydrate foods, even if the focus is not on carbohydrate restriction, specifically.

There's a lot more to cholesterol than just what we eat too. Case in point: when I was in school, an instructor told us about a study published several years earlier, but I don't recall the source. According to her report, a drug manufacturer was preparing a group of laboratory rabbits for testing a new anti-cholesterol drug. There were actually three groups of these rabbits. All of them were fed diets that normally create high cholesterol levels in that particular breed of rabbit. Just prior to the time scheduled to begin the drug testing, all the rabbits' blood was tested to make sure their cholesterol levels were actually high enough to run the tests. But one group out of the three consistently did not have high cholesterol levels. This baffled the researchers. All the rabbits were fed identical diets and had identical living conditions. So how could this be? They were at a complete loss for an explanation.

However, further investigation revealed that the group that had the lower cholesterol levels were housed in cages that were at eye level to the caretakers. When the rabbit feeders came around to feed them, they would take these rabbits out, love them and pet them. This was the only difference.

Researchers then tried doing the same thing with test rabbits at some other universities (taking one group out, loving and petting them) and they found similar, low-cholesterol results. So another way to keep your cholesterol levels down to a healthy level in a fun and exciting way is to have somebody you love "take you out of your cage" to love and be kind to you every day! (Reduce your stress!)

The most threatening cholesterol monsters we face in America today are stress and the combination of fats with carbohydrates – combinations such as the Great American staples: French fries, doughnuts, pasta and meatballs, steak and potatoes, bread and butter, ice cream, cookies, cakes, potato chips, and all manner of snacks. Eating fats without simultaneously consuming carbs is nowhere nearly as dangerous. But this ill-fated combination is a major harbinger of ill health and early death, particularly when combined with a high-stress lifestyle.

Since cardiovascular health is of such great concern to all diabetics, it's very important that you understand this subject so that you can avoid dangerous prescription drugs when possible and manage your health through natural, balanced means.

Protein – The Body's Building Blocks

I want to preface this section with my assurance that I have no bones to pick with people who choose to be vegetarians, either casually or as strict vegans. (Unless they're militantly browbeating me to join their ranks against my will.) We each have to choose for ourselves what works for us personally in terms of our beliefs, our life's philosophy, our personal health, our own spiritual convictions and our heredity.

I spent more than a year of my life as a vegetarian, so I've had that experience and I believe I gave it a truly fair trial. I have very good friends for whom it works much better than it did for me. They enjoy the vegetarian lifestyle and I do respect their choice as I do yours.

Protein is the subject of this chapter, however, and meat, of course, is the most bountiful source of complete proteins. Why do we need them? Everything in our bodies is made up of proteins and eating proteins gives us the complete compliment of essential amino acids. Amino acids are the building blocks we have to have in order to build the proteins necessary for all of our body processes.

Proteins are incredibly long, convoluted, complicated molecules, made from smaller, simpler molecules called amino acids. When proteins are digested and broken down into all of their components, including glucose and amino acids, the amino acids are taken inside the cells of our bodies to be used as building blocks. Those amino acid building blocks are then reassembled in specific sequences to build the required proteins. Proteins are what our muscles are made of as well as our connective tissue (like tendons, ligaments and bones) our hair and skin, our organs, our blood. Even our hormones contain proteins. Protein is the most vital player in every healing process in our bodies, especially after an injury.

Protein is so vital to our survival that if a person is starved of protein from other sources, the body will begin to break down its own protein to get the necessary amino acids to replenish the proteins that need replacing, inadequate as that process is. You've seen emaciated people like this in the pictures from the German, World War II concentration camps and some of the starving children in Africa.

There are 22 amino acids that make up proteins. Eight of them are called "essential amino acids" and the rest are termed "non-essential." Our bodies have the ability to make the fourteen non-essential amino acids on its own. But our bodies must obtain the eight essential amino acids from outside sources, in other words, from what we eat. If we're short on any of the amino acids, our bodies simply cannot manufacture all the healthy proteins it needs in order to maintain normal health and repair. This is an aspect that many who decide to become vegetarian, unfortunately, don't consider. Perhaps, they just don't fully understand how important this is. Getting a complete complement of amino acids requires a detailed knowledge of the amino acid content of foods, especially which amino acids are missing from which foods and how and where to get them. Often, to get all the required amino acids to make the proteins we have to have, a vegetarian has to eat certain foods together, like corn and beans or brown rice and beans. Each has some essential amino acids but not all of the necessary ones. Only by combining these foods, can the vegetarian get the full complement of amino acids we have to have to make the vital proteins we need to maintain good health.

All three of the above-mentioned foods have high carbohydrate content, however, so you can see that a type II diabetic who chooses to be a vegetarian faces some profound dietary challenges.

Another real problem faced by the vegetarian is how to get an adequate supply of vitamin B12 from nutritional sources. It's found almost exclusively in meat. If you're prone to select the vegetarian lifestyle for yourself, please do your due diligence. Study the literature and make sure you're getting all the amino acids you need in the right combinations on a daily basis and the other food requirements that may be lacking in an all-vegetable eating plan.

Supplement with vitamin B12 (regardless of the source), especially if your energy levels are low. B12 is the energy and stamina vitamin. Shortages of B12 can also make you vulnerable to homocysteine, a substance that's known to be a major player in the development of atherosclerosis (cardiovascular disease).

Protein is vital to the healing process after we've been injured. Whether the injury has been just a superficial trauma to the skin or a deeper injury involving muscle tissue or even our organs, protein is the major player contributing to our body's ability to make the appropriate repairs.

It's imperative to make a point here that few people ever consider. The trauma of surgery is no different, as far as your body is concerned, than being torn open by an assailant's knife, having your body ripped open by a chunk of jagged metal in a car accident, or having an organ torn out of your body by a piece of flying shrapnel from an exploding bomb! There may be differences in the cleanliness aspects of these injuries, how neatly the cuts were made, and the psychological effects that they have on us, but the body's repair mechanisms still only recognize that it has been profoundly torn open and it must repair itself in the very same way.

Protein is the primary building block for making those repairs since every tissue in the human body is made from proteins. So, after any injury, including surgery, to maximize the healing process, be sure to include adequate amounts of protein in your diet; or to be even more proactive, increase your protein intake to levels beyond what might otherwise be considered merely "adequate." This is particularly important to diabetics, since poor healing is a common symptom in both types of diabetes.

What might an "adequate" amount of protein be? Professional bodybuilders can give us some useful insight here. The process of competitive body building involves repeatedly over-working the muscles to the point that they start to break down and sustain microscopic injury. Then the bodybuilder allows time for "recovery" (the healing process). During that time, he or she eats proteins to maximize that repair process and minimize healing time. Then the bodybuilder goes through that whole process again and again on a regular basis.

Examining the protein intake of professional bodybuilders during this kind of training can, therefore, give us a good indicator of what may be an optimum regular protein intake for optimum healing after we sustain an injury or undergo surgery.

In one very informative book called, *"Get The Pump,"* written by a consortium of eight of America's most winning body building champions, the authors recommend eating at least 1.5 grams of protein in the daily diet for every pound of body weight. So, if a person weighs 150 pounds, for instance, according to their recommendation, he or she would need to consume 225 grams of protein daily. For a 200 pound person, 300 grams would be optimum. And, just in case you've forgotten your conversion tables, there are 28 grams in an ounce. Three hundred grams would therefore be between 10 and 11 ounces of protein for the day.

This isn't to say that if you eat these (adequate) amounts of proteins, you'll automatically put on massive muscle volume, not by a long shot! Believe me, most body builders only wish that it were that simple! It only means that you'll be sure to provide yourself with enough protein and you can have the confidence that your body can make the appropriate repairs whenever you're injured or have had a recent surgery.

Another thing you should be aware of is that simply consuming adequate amounts of protein is no guarantee that your body will actually be able to digest it and break it down into its component amino acids for you to be able to use. Proper food combining is an important aspect in maximizing your body's ability to use the foods you eat, including protein.

Protein must be exposed to a heavily acid environment in order to break down those incredibly long, convoluted molecules into their amino acid building blocks. The only environment in the human body with sufficient acid to break those proteins down is found in the stomach. Even in that harsh, acidic environment, according to Harvey and Marilyn Diamond, authors of the internationally acclaimed book, *"Fit For Life,"* it can take proteins from six to eight hours to be digested well enough to be properly absorbed through the intestines and into the body. And any dilution of the acid in the stomach only impairs complete digestion of the proteins.

This very important acid environment in the stomach can often be compromised by antacids like Tums or Rolaids, any of those "purple pills" that are supposed to be so great for chronic indigestion, by improper food combining, insufficient nerve flow to the stomach's acid-secreting lining or excess fluid consumption with meals.

So let's contrast protein digestion with carbohydrate digestion. Carbohydrates, unlike proteins, require an alkaline environment to be broken down into their component molecules. This is just the opposite of an acid environment such as we find inside of the stomach. The part of the digestive tract that provides this alkaline environment is the duodenum. This is the very first part of the small intestine, just beyond the stomach. I mention this so you'll have the groundwork to understand the process that I'm about to describe, the concept on which the book, *"Fit For Life,"* was based.

When we eat a piece of steak, for instance, the stomach recognizes it as protein and sends messages to the nervous system to keep the protein there in the stomach for six to eight hours – in an acid environment – so that it can let its acid break down the proteins for adequate digestion.

On the other hand, if we should eat a potato, the stomach would recognize the presence of the carbohydrates and send a message to the nervous system that would cause the lower valve of the stomach, the pyloric valve, to open after only a short time. The carbohydrates would pass into the duodenum so that they can be digested properly in that alkaline environment.

But, if we eat both a steak and a potato together, the nervous system gets mixed messages. The acid environment in the stomach gets diluted due to the presence of the carbohydrates. When the stomach senses the carbohydrates, it sends its message to open the pyloric valve earlier than it would have if it were just protein in the stomach. So the entire contents of the stomach; protein, carbohydrates and all, are passed into the duodenum, quite prematurely as far as protein digestion is concerned. So even if the person has eaten adequate amounts of protein, only a partially digested form of it is passed into the intestines and what is passed on is in a state that's impossible for the intestines to absorb as useable nutritional components. Instead, the protein remains in the intestines as an undigested, rotting glob of meat, with bacterial actions creating toxins along the way, and is eventually excreted, wasted.

At the same time, since the stomach did indeed recognize the presence of the protein, it did pour out lots of acid into the stomach for protein digestion. But because the presence of the carbohydrates caused the contents of the stomach to be passed along too soon, the acid still present from the stomach neutralizes so much of the alkaline contents of the duodenum that it renders the duodenum somewhat useless in digesting the carbohydrates.

So not only does the protein being passed along remain undigested, so do the carbohydrates! The result is a partially digested collection of putrefied "garbage" passing along through the intestines on which the natural bacteria in your intestines feed. The bacteria produce gas and toxins which are then absorbed through the intestinal walls into the blood stream! They also produce foul-smelling stools, not to mention insufficient nutrition.

Let's recap some basic food-combining guidelines developed by Dr. Herbert Sheldon in Texas in the 1940's and further developed by the Diamonds, mentioned above. Eat proteins alone or with salads. If carbohydrates absolutely must be included in the meal, be sure to make them very low-carb vegetables.

Eat bread, potatoes or high carb vegetables with salads. But refrain from eating high protein foods and high-carb foods together. For instance, avoid eating a steak and a potato. Have the steak with a salad or a potato with a salad, but avoid the steak with a potato. Actually, if you're a type II diabetic, avoid the potatoes and medium to high glycemic index carbohydrate foods altogether!

According to the food combining experts, it takes fruits, which are very high-carb foods, about a half an hour to move out of your stomach. It takes complex carbohydrates (like pasta, grains or potatoes) about two hours to get out of your stomach. It takes proteins about six to eight hours to move out of your stomach. This gives us a timeline for determining how long we should wait after eating proteins or carbs before we eat something else if we want to enjoy maximum digestive abilities. Wait thirty minutes after eating fruit before eating anything else. Wait about two hours after eating more complex carbohydrates before eating protein. Wait for six to eight hours after eating a protein meal before eating carbohydrates again.

If you're a type II diabetic, it's a good idea to restrict your carbs as much as possible anyway, having meals of proteins, fats and very low-carbohydrate, high-fiber content foods. Even though *"Fit For Life"* by Harvey and Marilyn Diamond may be a good reference for learning about efficient, healthy food combining, they recommend eating carbs for breakfast and lunch. That may be great for normally healthy people; however, if you're a type II diabetic or pre-diabetic – DON'T! This book is recommended only for the purpose of understanding food combining principles. It is *not* recommended as a complete eating plan for type II diabetics!

I wanted to mention again that the purple pills (Nexium and Prilosec, for instance) inhibit your body's ability to digest proteins. Why? Because, as you just saw, proteins require an acid environment for adequate digestion. These drugs, both the prescription forms and the over-the-counter kinds, work by decreasing the production of adequate amounts of acid in the stomach. Without that adequate stomach acid, your body can't break down protein nor will it be able to absorb the calcium in your foods or supplements.

In my opinion as a doctor of chiropractic, if you suffer from reflux, it's far more desirable to restore normal nerve function to the valves in the stomach, especially the top one – the cardiac valve – by spinal manipulation, so that the valve functions like it's supposed to. This tends to keep the acid in the stomach where it's supposed to be so it can digest the food rather than destroying this vital digestive solution. In terms of long-term health and longevity, this is certainly far better than destroying the stomach's ability to digest protein by using either prescription or over-the-counter drugs. If you suffer from chronic indigestion or acid reflux ("disease"), also known as GERD or GIRD, ask your chiropractor to evaluate your "T5 and T6." These are the fifth and sixth vertebrae in the center of your back. These are where nerves that control the stomach exit from the spine. Also have him or her check C1 (the first cervical vertebra at the top of your neck). Misalignments at C1 can affect the Vagus nerve which can, in turn, affect the operation of the stomach.

B. I. was in his mid twenties when he first became a patient with low back pains. During the initial work-up he also mentioned that he suffered from gastric reflux. So I paid special attention to his mid back during my examinations and discovered misalignments at T5 and T6 and corrected them. I explained to him how those specific spinal misalignments were related to his reflux and heartburn.

At his next visit, he reported that his reflux had not given him any problems since the adjustment. Over the past decade, when he does experience infrequent heartburn (perhaps 1-3 times a year) he presents for an adjustment and enjoys months of symptom -free GI function.

The same warning that applies for the purple pills obviously holds true for antacids. They work by neutralizing stomach acid, destroying the necessary pH levels and making the stomach more alkaline, thus inhibiting protein digestion.

An acid environment is also required in the stomach for the body to absorb calcium and use it. Otherwise the calcium just passes through the digestive system and is excreted. So taking Tums, or any antacid, as a calcium source will practically guarantee that you will *not* be able to absorb the calcium in it. Just the fact that it's an antacid means that it will neutralize the stomach acid and the calcium simply cannot be absorbed.

To re-cap:

We have to have protein for the body to be able to re-build and repair itself daily.

Eight of the 22 amino acids which are the building blocks for proteins, must come from what we eat. They're called "essential amino acids."

Vegetarian diets must be thoroughly researched and planned if the vegetarian hopes to get all of the necessary amino acids in the right combinations and sufficient amounts of vitamin B12 to maintain health and the body's ability to heal itself.

An adequate amount of daily protein could be established by following the research of bodybuilders – eat at least 1.5 grams of protein for every pound of body weight you carry. (There are 28 grams in an ounce.)

Simply eating the right amounts of protein will not assure us that we will be able to digest and absorb the amounts of amino acids that we must have. Proper, complete digestion is a vital player for optimum health, so we should always take the necessary steps to maximize the efficiency of our digestive processes.

Several things can impede the digestive process; most importantly, improper food combining, those "purple pills" and antacids.

The simplest rule for food combining is to eat proteins and carbohydrates separately, at different meals. Wait six hours after eating protein to eat carbohydrates. Wait two hours after eating carbs to eat protein.

If you're a type II diabetic, stay away from the carbohydrates as much as you can.

"Hay," What About Fiber?

Dietary fiber is very important and there's a lot of information in the mainstream media about it – in magazines, newspapers, talk shows. Most of it's true and logical. But, although the majority of the popular information about fiber may work out for some people, some of it simply doesn't apply, at least to some diabetics. Unfortunately, some information can even prove to be quite harmful, especially for the type II diabetic. Not all bodies are the same and you'll be able to prove that to yourself with your daily testing. We'll go over those testing procedures in much more detail later in this book.

First, let's look at some of the more universal benefits of fiber. Primarily, fiber is indigestible, which ironically offers us one of its greatest benefits. Eating fiber is kind of like chewing up and swallowing wood. These woody little fiber molecules are basically the same as some sugar or other carbohydrate molecules, except that they're shaped somewhat differently. It's that slight difference in the shape of the molecule that makes fiber impossible for humans to digest. Our bodies don't recognize it as a food nor do they have the enzymes needed to digest it, so our bodies can't break it down into its simple components of glucose, carbon dioxide and water. We simply pass the fiber through our systems, more or less in its original form.

If we can't digest it, then why on earth would fiber be such a good thing for us to eat? Because it's this very quality of indigestibility that gives it value. One of the most important qualities of fiber is its ability to attract, absorb and hold water. When we have chewed-up fiber in our digestive tract, it does just that. It attracts, absorbs and holds water, which, in turn, keeps our stools soft and moist. That keeps bowel movements easy and prevents constipation. And since it attaches to cholesterol, fiber also serves as sort of a "broom" to "sweep" the colon clean.

Without adequate fiber, the food passing through the digestive tract can therefore become too dry, making the stools that pass through it dry and hard – prime contributors to chronic constipation, hemorrhoids and colon cancer. The American diet, which is typically sorely lacking in adequate amounts of water and fiber, adds significantly to the danger of long-term or frequent constipation. So you can understand why fiber is such a vital part of the daily diet for a healthy colon.

Please allow me to digress for a few paragraphs to emphasize some points about water. It's very important to understand that soft drinks, tea, coffee or fruit juices, don't count as water. It's absolutely vital to understand this point. In fact, for every ounce of soft drinks or coffee that you do drink, you should drink that much more water that day to dilute their effects. A healthy human body is more than 95 percent water. Dehydration contributes significantly to a plethora of human ailments.

How much water is enough? Research published in the form of an amazing book called, *"Your Body's Many Cries For Water,"* by Dr. F. Batmanghelidj suggests that we need a half an ounce of water every day for every pound of body weight. So if you weigh 150 pounds, you'd need seventy-five ounces of water daily. The old suggestion that you drink eight, 8-ounce glasses of water daily (sixty-four ounces) would be the right amount for people who weighed how much? That's right only 128 pounds! That may have been a good ball-park, generalized figure for the public at large in 1945 when that was much closer to the average weight of Americans; however that hasn't been anywhere near the average weight for us now for dozens of years.

Divide your weight by two. That's how much water you need in ounces every day. Tea doesn't count, nor does juice, not coffee, not soft drinks – only water. It can be spring water, reverse-osmosis drinking water, even tap water in some places. But it must be water!

There's controversy about drinking distilled water however because it can leach out our minerals. Other researchers tell us that using distilled water is fine if you add about a teaspoon of sea salt to each gallon to replace the natural minerals.

If you just can't stand drinking water by itself, squeeze one slice of lemon into it. The lemon slice is good for neutralizing the chlorine in tap water too. In most places, bottled water is tastier than tap water. But be sure to get your water in adequate amounts.

Back to the benefits of fiber. Fiber also binds to bile salts in the intestines. Bile is manufactured in the liver for the purpose of breaking down and digesting the fats that we eat. During the digestion process, bile is converted to bile salts. These bile salts are actually toxic, so if they stay in the digestive tract too long they can cause intestinal problems. They can also be absorbed into the body where they may stress internal organs as well. When the fiber binds to bile salts in the digestive tract, it helps to neutralize their effects, and the presence of the fiber keeps food in the digestive tract moving along through the intestines without the delays of constipation. Keeping the contents moving through the intestines is important so that the bile salts will not release toxins into the blood stream through the intestinal walls.

Toxicity from the bile salts is reputed to be a contributor to colon cancer. Adequate fiber in the daily diet, on the other hand, is famous for its anti-colon cancer benefits.

Where do we get fiber? We get it from just about any kind of vegetable matter. Some vegetables certainly have higher fiber content than others. For instance, I was surprised to discover that an avocado contains more fiber than the average bran muffin! Salads are an excellent source of fiber as well as one of the healthiest. Nuts and seeds are also high in fiber. The Abbreviated Carbohydrate Chart in the back of this book notes the grams of fiber contained in the foods that are listed there.

One of the potential dangers that people encounter when they embark on a low-carbohydrate diet is a lack of fiber. Meat doesn't have fiber, nor does fat. In their efforts to avoid carbohydrates, people often limit their food intake to these non-fiber foods and suffer from sluggish digestion, constipation and all the health challenges that they bring with them.

True, the only three categories of human nutrients are protein (like meats), fats (including oils) and carbohydrates. It seems perfectly logical at first, then, that if you want to limit your consumption of carbohydrates, the only two things left for us to eat would be meat and fats. But that assumption would reflect a lack of understanding of the role of fiber or where it comes from. I know that this may be getting a bit confusing, but please bear with me. Even though there are only three actual nutrients – protein, fat and carbohydrates – that's not all we eat. The other thing we eat, which is NOT a nutrient – because we can't digest it – is fiber.

So, how does fiber fit into the overall dietary picture in a restricted carbohydrate diet? We know that plants are our source for fiber. But we also know that plants are our sources of carbohydrates. The two molecules, carbohydrates and fiber, are very similar but one can be digested (carbohydrates) and the other can't (the fiber). If we want to limit our carbohydrates, the question we have to address is, "How do we get enough fiber without getting excess carbs too?"

The good news is that some plants have almost no carbohydrates at all. The bad news is that other plants have lots of carbs. Bananas and pineapples, for instance, may have plenty of fiber but they're also very high in sugars (concentrated carbohydrates) even for fruits. All fruits are high in carbohydrates.

Peas, carrots, sweet potatoes, yams, potatoes, and beans, even though they may have adequate amounts of fiber, are nonetheless high in carbohydrates as well.

Salad greens, spinach, celery and radishes, on the other hand, have negligible amounts of carbohydrates, but are indeed high in fiber. Nuts and seeds are high in fiber, but they have varying concentrations of carbohydrate content. Which particular nuts and seeds our bodies can tolerate as type II diabetics will vary from person to person.

If you have type II diabetes, and you're making an effort to control it with a restricted carbohydrate intake (which I believe is the ideal method), it's very important for you to discover which high fiber, low carbohydrate vegetable sources you can safely enjoy and include plenty of those foods in your daily diet. Twenty-five grams of fiber per day is a typical minimum daily recommendation.

There is one particular bit of information about fiber that you'll read in various publications, or even hear from doctors, nurses and nutritionists (if you haven't already) that could actually be harmful to you if you're a type II diabetic. There's a theory in popular nutrition circles that a person can consume carbohydrates in combination with fiber and for every gram of fiber you're consuming, you can completely avoid all of the effects of that same amount of carbohydrates. You see this on labeling everywhere, especially on the snack foods. These labels pronounce in big, bold letters, "Only 3 grams net carbs!" The red-lights-and-sirens warning here for the carbohydrate sensitive person (the type II diabetic) is the word buried right in the center of the proclamation – that little word "net." Any time you see the word "net" before the word carbohydrates, it means that the labeler has used this popular method of calculating the carbohydrates. That is to say that they have determined the actual carbohydrate content of servings in the package, subtracted the fiber content per serving and then proudly labeled the difference as "Net Carbs." But packaging laws, thankfully, still require them to put the actual, full carbohydrate content onto the back of the package.

For instance, I've picked up several "low carb" snack bars in the grocery store which were labeled as only containing two or three "net" carbs, but the labeling on the back of the package showed that there were actually more than twenty grams of carbohydrates in the food! They were supposed to be canceled out by the presence of several grams of fiber.

Wanting desperately to believe that my wife could really eat one of these luscious goodies with no more consequence than two or three carbohydrates would normally cause, we've tried them. But to date, in each case, subsequent testing of the blood sugar and the urine has shown responses identical to an intake of over twenty grams of pure, raw, unadulterated carbohydrates from any high-carb food. Regardless of the "NET" figure advertised, the actual effects on her blood sugar, and my own, have been in proportion to the actual full carbohydrate content of the food, regardless of the theoretically canceling effects of the fiber!

This leaves me to question much of the "net carb" theory. For instance, what specific effects is the fiber truly supposed to be canceling? Is it supposed to be in terms of blood sugar readings or some other effect? Because in the case of both my wife and myself, that theory has proven to be unreliable in terms of measured blood sugar effects. I can only assume that if it's true for us, it must be true for a great many type II diabetics and pre-diabetics as well.

Maybe the effect measured by the "net carb" theory is a measure of some other physiological phenomenon. But the most important thing in the context of this book is that the concept of "net carbs" can't always be trusted as true in terms of blood sugar in type II diabetics and pre-diabetics, despite the popular hopes and assumptions.

In all fairness, I haven't tried it with a large cross-section of diabetics to see if other type II diabetics like my wife and pre-diabetics like myself are all as sensitive to carbohydrates as we are, even in the presence of fiber. But I certainly expect it to be true for very many, if not the majority.

If you want to experiment with this idea yourself (and I recommend that you do), instead of just taking my word for it or risking your life on the sales desires of snack food manufacturers, use your own blood glucose meter. You can buy them readily and without a prescription at any drug store. Test your blood when you first arise each morning, for a week. Test again about two hours after a breakfast of bacon and eggs, but without toast, without juice, or other carbs every day during the same week. Make sure your breakfast is all protein and fats – no carbs. Coffee or tea is fine, with heavy cream if you like, and possibly some Sweet & Low or Stevia. This will give you a baseline average reading on your glucose meter for later comparison. Write down your numbers and take an average for the week.

Then for breakfast one morning, include one or two pieces of toast. Look on the bread label to see what the actual carbohydrate content of each slice is. A slice of bread has an average of from 12 to 21 grams of carbohydrates depending on a number of factors. For this part of your experiment, you should be consuming about 21 grams of carbohydrates in your toasted bread. Then, note the reading on your meter, testing two hours after breakfast. It should be noticeably higher.

The next morning, instead of the toast, include one of the "low carb" snack bars with a low number of "net carbs" on the front label but with about 21 grams of actual carbs on the back label. Again, test with your meter two hours after you eat and note that reading. If this reading for the snack bar is similar to the breakfast that included toast, you know that the "net carb" theory doesn't work for you either. If this is the case for you, you'll always have to look at that actual carbohydrate content on the back of labels and disregard the "net carbs" advertising on the fronts of packages.

A note of caution – some type II diabetics don't register the effects of carb loading for 36 to 48 hours, so the above testing may need to be altered to reflect this if you discover that you fall into that category.

This "net carb" labeling is not limited to snack bars either. I've seen it on ice cream, frozen dinners, desserts and boxed foods as well. If you truly want to achieve maximum health despite your type II diabetes, *you must become a master at reading and interpreting labels.* You should also memorize the true carbohydrate content of foods that have no labels, such as fresh vegetables.

As another short aside, in regard to labeling, "no sugar added" or "sugar free" do not mean low carbohydrate content, necessarily. Always be sure to look at the label to discover the actual content of carbohydrates in the food and never make assumptions.

To recap, fiber is a vital consumable that's not actually a food because it's impossible to digest. Its presence in our digestive tract keeps its contents moist, soft and moving through the intestines at a normal rate. Because of its ability to soften stools, to keep our food moving through our digestive tract at a reasonable rate and to bind to bile salts, it's a valuable dietary component for preventing constipation and cancers in the digestive tract. So it's incredibly important!

Vegetables, fruits and nuts are our sources of fiber. We have to learn which ones are high in fiber but very low in carbohydrates. These are the preferred ones we should include in our daily diets if we're type II diabetics or pre-diabetics. We must include lots of these vegetables in our daily diets and minimize or eliminate the ones that are higher in carbohydrates.

The term, "net carbs," just means the number of grams of actual carbohydrates per serving minus the number of grams of fiber. This is not necessarily of any useful consequence in terms of its effects on blood sugar in type II diabetics or pre-diabetics. If you think you want to try these low "net carb" foods, it's absolutely essential that you know exactly how they're going to affect your own personal blood sugar levels by testing with your own blood glucose meter. Your personal carbohydrate/insulin metabolism may very well disagree with the labeling people.

"People's bodies don't read the books," my instructors used to say, meaning that regardless of what's in the books, people's bodies are individual and simply can't be generalized. What's true in even a majority of cases may not be true for everybody. And if you're one of the people for whom one of these assumed "truths" does not apply, it matters very little what others consider those generalized "truths" to be.

The bottom line is that you must determine what YOUR body does with carbohydrates when it's combined with fiber. If the "net" carb hypothesis actually works for you and helps you to control your own, personal blood sugar levels, by all means enjoy yourself. But you will never know if that's the case if you don't test it on your own metabolism.

The Glycemic Index

It just naturally should follow that a chapter subsequent to one on fiber would be a chapter about the glycemic index. The subject doesn't quite fit into a discussion on fiber, but some of the arguments are similar – "good carbs/bad carbs/net carbs," etc. The glycemic index supporters maintain that the slower carbohydrates are delivered into your system, the better off you'll be. That's certainly true for healthy people, but if you have type II diabetes it's a dangerous over-simplification. All carbohydrates deliver concentrated glucose into the blood stream too quickly for the type II diabetic to handle. That's why they have type II diabetes!

What is the glycemic index? It's a ranking of foods containing carbohydrates based on their immediate effects on your blood sugar. Carbohydrates that break down into glucose the fastest have the highest glycemic index numbers. The blood sugar response is quick and high. Carbs from foods that break down more slowly release glucose more gradually into the blood stream. They have lower glycemic index numbers.

While those who espouse the glycemic index paradigm speak in terms of "good carbs" and "bad carbs," they don't seem to truly understand the process of the development of type II diabetes as opposed to type I and the role of all carbohydrates for the intermediate to advanced type II diabetic. Most carbs are poison for the type II diabetic even if some are more harmful than others. All carbs release their glucose into the blood stream within about two hours - too quickly.

I must admit that, according to my understanding of the glycemic index, following it would probably be a great preventative eating consideration for people who think they might be at risk for developing type II diabetes, but who are not yet either diabetic or pre-diabetic (hyperinsulinemic). These would include those people who have a family history of type II diabetes and people who find themselves gaining weight very easily. However, I also believe that once a person's metabolism has developed into a pre-diabetic condition in which the pancreas has already been trained to over react as a course of habit to the presence of even complex carbohydrates, suddenly adopting the recommendations of a low glycemic index diet would be "closing the barn door after the horse got out," simply too little too late.

For instance, low glycemic index diet plans recommend that you "use breakfast cereals based on oats, barley and bran." But as I explain throughout this book, these are grains that are typically high enough in carbohydrate content to easily push type II diabetics into excreting sugar in their urine and pushing their blood sugar levels uncomfortably, or even dangerously, high. Later in this book, you'll also read about the undesirable role of grains in precipitating joint pains.

Low glycemic index eating plans also typically include recommendations to "use 'grainy' breads made with whole seeds." I agree that if a type II diabetic were to break down and submit to the very unhealthy temptation of eating a piece of bread, this might be the bread of choice, but as I've explained in several places in this text, bread should simply be considered poison for most type II diabetics because of its invariable and immediate effects on blood sugar. If you're not a type II diabetic or pre-diabetic, these breads might be a great recommendation. But it's certainly not healthy for the people for whom this book is written.

Those who embrace the glycemic index as a guide for nutrition recommend that you "reduce the amount of potatoes you eat" and to "enjoy all types of fruit and vegetables." Please refer to the chapter on The Food Pyramids. If you follow their advice to eat any potatoes at all, vegetables like carrots, tomatoes, peas or other high-carb vegetables, or fruits - always high-carbohydrate foods, your blood sugar can skyrocket if you're a type II diabetic! These foods are simply dangerous in any amounts for type II diabetics. They contribute to the problem rather than to any alleviation of the problem. In fact, over time, they'll make it even worse.

Understanding the glycemic index can, however, give you some insight into the degree of undesirability of foods that do contain carbohydrates. The higher the glycemic index number of a carbohydrate-containing food, the more damaging it will be for the type II diabetic. So if you have access to a glycemic index chart for foods, you can use it to make sure that the vegetables, fruits and nuts that you choose are in the lowest possible ranking of the index – the ones that will cause you the least harm.

The higher the index number, the higher the carbohydrate content, the higher the carbohydrate concentration in the food, the more rapidly the blood sugar rises in response and thus, the more overwhelming the corresponding insulin response, continuing to worsen the development of type II diabetes.

However, staying with foods in the range of the very lowest numbers on the glycemic index is said to help your body's cells to become more sensitive to insulin over time. And if type II diabetics absolutely must have carbohydrate foods, they certainly should be ones that are very low on the glycemic index.

If you decide to choose your foods based on the glycemic index, it is still vitally important for you to know the exact effects that those foods will have on YOUR body, not just some hypothetical, generic chart. Use your urine testing sticks (see the chapter on Testing) and your glucose meter to measure the actual numbers that your food choices produce in your own, individual system in terms of blood sugar and sugar in the urine. The entire reason for staying with foods with a low glycemic index is to control your blood sugar. Don't rely on anybody's theories *or any research that was performed on healthy people without type II diabetes, or on mixed groups of both type II and type I diabetics!* Get your own numbers rather than gambling with your health and your life.

A second term you'll find relating to the glycemic index is "glycemic load." It's calculated by multiplying the glycemic index number by the grams of carbs per serving of the food in question.

A unit of glycemic load is about equal to the effect of one gram of glucose. The glycemic index database gives both the glycemic index and the glycemic load.

Whether you decide to measure your carbohydrate intake by grams on the package or by the glycemic index, be sure to keep a close count on what amounts of carbs you're consuming and what their effects are on your own, personal metabolism. Nobody, including healthcare professionals, will be able to manage your blood sugar as well as you can yourself.

Exercise: Use It Or Lose It

So often we hear that we should, "Eat right and exercise," to get healthy and stay that way. When I hear this, all I can do is chuckle. As sound as that advice may be, defining exactly what it means is an incredibly monstrous task to tackle. Let's look at "eating right:" What about cholesterol? (A gross misunderstanding, at best, as you read earlier in this book.) What about the food pyramid? (If you follow that mistaken concept, you're almost guaranteed to become overweight, develop Osteoarthritis and degenerate into type II diabetes if you have any proclivity toward it at all.) What about avoiding meat? (Do this and you cheat yourself out of vitamin B12 and the valuable protein building blocks your body requires to heal from injuries and to rebuild itself on a daily basis.) What about including lots of whole grains and pasta in your diet? I personally believe that this is one of the greatest nutritional contributors to both the pain in all forms of arthritis and to obesity in both people and pets in America.

So, "Eat right?" What does that mean? I hope that former sections of this book have given you some useful insight into some aspects of that subject. More will be given later. Now for exercise.

Do we walk for three miles a day? Do we lift weights three times a week? Do we attend aerobics classes? Yoga? Pilates? What might, "Exercise," mean?

The scientific literature describes something called "Wolfe's Law," referring to human physiology (how the body works). You've probably heard this law reduced to a very simple sentence – "Use it or lose it." In a nutshell, that describes Wolfe's Law very well. For instance, you've seen people who were paralyzed from the waist down and who had been confined to a wheelchair for a long time. You may have noticed that their legs became very thin from a process called "atrophy" or "muscle wasting." The muscles aren't being used, so they begin to disappear. Use it or lose it!

You may have been in great shape at one time in your life, perhaps in high school or in college, but now may find that you're not able to meet many of the physical challenges you easily met on a regular basis back then. You're "out of training." Being out of training causes you to lose stamina and strength. Use it or lose it!

One of the things now recommended for senior citizens in order to sharpen their mental skills is to do crossword puzzles or to study a foreign language. The mind is apparently just like our muscles. It has to be exercised too in order to remain strong, supple and durable. Use it or lose it!

Osteoporosis is a big concern for post-menopausal women in our country. So women are gobbling down tons of calcium and/ or prescription drugs in a completely misinformed and extremely limited attempt to counteract it. The mere act of swallowing calcium will not necessarily get it into your bones! You have to give the bones a reason to take it in and a way to make that happen. The one and only reason a bone takes in more calcium is the stress of using the bone – exercise! Without exercise, the calcium is totally useless in terms of bone strength and, in fact may only result in dry, flaky, cracking skin especially around the backs of your heels. In truth, there are very few Americans who actually lack sufficient calcium in their diets. Your body will also need adequate amounts of vitamin D, (you can get that from sunshine) and natural progesterone to most effectively combat Osteoporosis. (For more on this subject, pick up a copy of, *"What Your Doctor May Not Tell You About Menopause,"* by Dr. John R Lee.)

Exercising, (preferably in the sun so the body can produce its own vitamin D) is one of the most important factors for keeping your bones strong and helping to replace bone loss. Use it or lose it!

A little more about Vitamin D: it's needed for calcium to get into the bone matrix. Without it you can eat all the calcium in the world and it'll never make it into your bones. The very best and safest source of Vitamin D is exposure to sunshine. According to research by Dr. David Williams, publisher of *"Alternatives,"* one should get exposure to sunshine daily, but not enough to turn your skin pink, and it should be WITHOUT sunscreen.

Sunscreen contains up to five different cancer-causing chemicals, especially para-aminobenzoic acid (PABA), the chemical hailed most for its sun screening qualities. The other four to look for: benzophenone -3 (Bp-3), homosalate (HMS), octyl-methoxycinnamate (OMC) and 4-methyl-benzylidene camphor (4-MBC).

Vitamin D deficiencies have also been linked to glucose intolerance, degenerative vascular disease, high blood pressure and depression. All four of these symptoms are typically associated with diabetes.

So the very first argument for exercising regularly is to make sure that we'll be able continue to move about, to work, to play and to have our bodies continue to function the way they were designed to function. "Use it or lose it," Wolfe's Law.

As well as protecting us from losing functions and vital tissue, exercise accomplishes several other benefits which would be difficult to accomplish by any other means. For instance, it boosts the effectiveness of two separate circulation systems in the body: blood circulation and lymphatic circulation.

The lymphatic system is a labyrinth of channels with filters that runs alongside the circulatory system. It circulates a substance called interstitial fluid through the lymph nodes throughout the body. These lymph nodes remove and destroy microorganisms and microscopic particles that shouldn't be there. This is why we get swollen "glands" when we're sick or have an infection. They're not really glands at all, but lymph nodes swollen with bacteria, viruses and/or fungi. This system is considered a very important component of our immune systems.

But the lymphatic system has no separate pump of its own to keep the fluid circulating like the circulatory system has a heart to pump our blood. The only way that the fluid can be circulated through the lymphatic system is with exercise, the contracting and relaxing of our muscles which in turn pushes the fluid along its course.

Circulating our blood is not as easy as we might assume either. You might think that just getting the heart rate up would be enough to keep the blood circulating at optimum levels but that's actually only half of the picture. The heart pumps out high oxygen-content, red blood through the arteries quite well. But once the blood is squeezed through the tiny capillaries at the ends of the arteries and arterioles, it has lost a lot of the heart's pressure and thus its ability to continue through the system. So the veins, the blood vessels that carry high carbon dioxide-content, purple blood back to the heart, have anti-back-flow valves along their entire length that keep the blood from flowing backward against the intended flow. These valves keep the blood flowing in one direction, back toward the heart. However, the pumping action of the heart is still poorly felt in the veins. Fortunately for us, the blood can be squeezed through the veins just like we squeeze toothpaste through a tube. Every time we tighten a muscle, the veins within that muscle are squeezed. When the veins are squeezed, because of the anti-back-flow valves, the blood can only go in one direction – toward the heart. The value of this muscle-assisted pumping action on the blood flow can't be overstated!

Congestive heart failure is a prime example of this process not working as it should. The heart is like any other muscle. It even takes the, "use it or lose it," concept one step further and actually works against us. We know that when we don't use a muscle, it shrinks – atrophies. Conversely, when we work a muscle very hard, it grows bigger. When we're inactive, we don't have the benefit of the pumping action of the muscles throughout our bodies to get the blood back to the heart through the veins. Therefore, the heart has to do all the work. So it must work harder to get the blood all the way through the system. This extra work (increased blood pressure) over time causes the heart muscle to get bigger and bigger. This results in the infamous "enlargement of the heart." The problem with this condition is that not only does the heart enlarge on the outside, it also enlarges on the inside. This leaves less empty volume inside the heart for the blood to fill and then be pumped out to the body. The blood becomes more and more difficult for the heart to pump through the system and the cycle just snowballs. Eventually, the heart becomes incapable of doing its job and the blood backs up in the venous part of the circulatory system. Eventually, the heart exhausts and simply stops – congestive heart failure.

Distinct symptoms are evident as congestive heart failure develops. The person may often get short of breath and the extremities (arms and legs) swell with fluid. A condition called "pitting edema" is one of the hallmarks of this swelling. Pitting edema is identified by pushing on the lower half of the shin with the point of a finger. If it makes a "pit," a deep indentation, and does not rebound quickly, that's known as pitting edema.

In the later stages of congestive heart failure, a person may even experience pneumonia-like symptoms like coughing and fluid in the lungs.

The best possible prevention for congestive heart failure is regular exercise in which you're contracting most of your body's muscles several times, repeatedly, in order to strongly pump the blood volume through the veins, back toward the heart taking some of the pressure off the cardiac muscle.

A good way to begin this kind of exercise is to aim for twenty minutes, three times weekly, doing whatever you enjoy that gets your heart rate to 120 if you're under 45, to 110 if you're between 45 and 60 or to 105 if you're over 60. It might be dancing, walking, calisthenics or whatever exercise you enjoy doing. These are general guidelines, however. Don't push yourself to getting very out of breath if you haven't exercised for some time. Work your way up to this if you must. Start slowly and progress a little at a time. In fact, I always recommend starting with the ridiculously easy and increasing it gradually from there.

For instance, if you're very out of shape and would like to start a walking routine, don't attempt to start by walking a mile out and a mile back. It would be self-defeating. Start by walking a block or a half a block or two houses down the block. When you feel really comfortable getting there and back on a regular basis, increase it a little. Continue adding distance only as you train for it.

In-flight venous thrombosis is a serious threat to health that has recently been in the news too. Officials have noticed an inordinate number of patients with dislodged venous thromboses (blood clots) who had recently experienced a long airline flight. Here's what happens: A person whose circulation isn't that great to begin with books a transcontinental flight, say from Los Angeles to Boston. During that time, he sits in his seat dutifully staying out of everybody's way and hardly moving at all. In other words, he doesn't contract any muscles to pump the blood through his veins. The slow-moving blood then forms a clot in one of his leg veins because it simply isn't moving well. Later, after the flight as he begins moving around again, the clot dislodges, travels to the heart and causes a heart attack or to the brain where it causes a stroke. This is a good reason to exercise your legs often before and during a flight. Also, walk when you can in the airports and be sure to move your legs frequently, tightening and relaxing the muscles, during all flights.

Exercise also creates more energy in your body on a regular basis. Inside your muscle cells are little "organelles," cell components that have specific functions inside the cell. Some build your proteins, some build your DNA and RNA, some are responsible for cell duplication, etc. Each has a specific function. One type of organelle is called a mitochondrion. Mitochondria are the organelles that turn your blood glucose (blood sugar) into energy – little "powerhouses" of your cells.

An interesting thing happens when we get into a regular exercise routine. The mitochondria, "realizing" that they need to produce more energy to meet the exercise demands, actually reproduce, creating extra numbers of mitochondria within the cells. When there are more mitochondria, more energy is produced – 24 hours a day. Also, more energy is used because it requires a certain amount of energy to produce those energy reserves. Your metabolism becomes more active, more efficient and you burn off more fat, *24 hours a day!*

So when people tell you that they can't exercise because they just don't have the energy, you now know that they're putting the cart before the horse. If you don't create a need in the body for energy, your body will decrease its production of energy. Use it or lose it! Initiating and maintaining a REGULAR exercise routine is one of the very best ways to create more consistent energy on a day to day basis over a long period of time.

And of particular interest to the type II diabetic is the phenomenon of exercise carrying glucose (blood sugar) into the cells. We've described the process of our cells becoming resistant to insulin during the development of type II diabetes as the body's way of preventing blood glucose crashes (hypoglycemia). One way to help overcome this resistance to insulin is through strenuous exercise. This is another fact that's well researched and proven by the professional body building community. Strenuous exercise depletes the glucose stores within the cells as it's used up for energy, which creates a new energy demand. This demand itself overcomes the cells' resistance temporarily and allows the insulin to carry the blood sugar out of the blood and into the cells where the need has been created. The blood sugar is decreased in a meaningful way, providing needed nutrition to the body's tissues instead of simply neutralizing the glucose and making it unavailable as happens with blood sugar-reducing drugs like Glucophage.

Exercise is preferred to Glucophage when possible because the way this drug brings down the blood sugar is by destroying it, making it not only disappear in the blood but also making it unavailable for normal nutrition and conversion into much needed energy that we can use for getting enough, life-giving exercise.

What kind of exercise is best? There are basically three categories to consider:

1) positional - such as yoga for flexibility,
2) aerobic - for maximum cardiac benefit and weight loss, and
3) resistance training - for muscle toning and developing more mitochondria in the muscles.

Yoga is recommended as the most beneficial type of exercise for fibromyalgia patients, according to the research in Leon Chaitow's book, *"Fibromyalgia Syndrome, A Practitioner's Guide to Treatment."* So if you suffer with chronic pain all over your body, this would probably be the best way to begin. This isn't standing on your head and doing impossible positions for hours, but gentle, specific positions called "postures" for maximizing your body's mobility and flexibility and learning how to master your breathing for maximum health benefits and pain relief.

Aerobic exercise is exercise that oxygenates your blood without creating an "oxygen deficit." When there's an excess demand for oxygen from exercise, called an oxygen deficit, that type of exercise is termed "anaerobic" exercise. The anaerobic form of exercise is the one that causes the soreness one feels after hard exercise. It makes you very hungry too. The soreness from anaerobic exercise is actually from the production of lactic acid, a by-product of burning fuels other than what your muscles have readily stored for that purpose.

Determining how to stay in the aerobic state and avoid the anaerobic state is actually pretty simple. As long as you can breathe easily, you are operating in the aerobic state. When you start to get out of breath, that indicates an oxygen deficit, signaling the entry into anaerobic exercise levels.

Aerobic exercise is what most exercise physiologists recommend for maximum cardiac benefit. It's also the best exercise range for losing weight. Because you never lose your breath, you can actually exercise for more extended periods, allowing you to burn off more calories. Good aerobic exercises for beginners include swimming, walking, mild dancing, golfing (especially when you walk the course instead of ride) and Tai Chi. The typical "aerobics" classes at your local gym are usually NOT aerobic at all unless you're 18 years old and extremely athletic already! Most people would have to have been doing aerobic exercises for years, stretching themselves to the point of getting out of breath for an extended training period to be able to participate in the typical aerobics class at the gym and still remain within the aerobic state. If this is your goal – to work out at the aerobics classes in the gym, you'll need to work up to it very slowly over a long period of time. Again, to keep yourself in the aerobic state, keep from getting out of breath. Once you get out of breath, you're in the anaerobic state and working against the benefits you're trying to achieve.

Resistance training is also known as weight training or weight lifting. This is actually the form of exercise that has the greatest potential for helping you reduce your blood sugar as a type II diabetic. I'm not recommending that you become a body builder because that's not really necessary. But to get the greatest benefit, you'll want to challenge yourself.

My best recommendation here is to find a personal trainer, usually available at any gym. Tell the trainer that you don't want to put on a lot of bulky muscles, but that you do want to tone the muscles that you have. Then, during your program, keep in mind that you want to stay in the aerobic range (not getting out of breath) for maximum benefits as a type II diabetic and adjust your workouts accordingly.

Ask your trainer to give you a variety of specific resistance exercises that take you to the point of fatigue by the third set of each exercise. Over a period of time, you'll need to increase the amount of weight to get you to that fatigue point as you get stronger. That and your increased energy and stamina levels will be how you'll know that your muscle cells are creating more mitochondria.

Be sure to tell your trainer that as a type II diabetic, you have very strict limitations on your carbohydrate intake and will NOT be able to follow his or her normal nutritional recommendations for a work-out regimen. *No carbs, no exceptions!*

If you have no trainer available or you're interested in more aggressive resistance training and true body shaping, I recommend subscribing to some of the body building magazines available at most news stands and supermarkets. After researching several of them for more than a year, I've been pleasantly surprised with the real, scientific research that's performed and referred to by most professional body builders. They, as a rule, have a great understanding of nutrition in a healthy person (not type II diabetics, however,) and know their exercise physiology extremely well, even if their exact opinions vary within the profession.

Whatever you decide to do for your regular exercise routine, the most important thing is that you do chose something. Choose a form of exercise that you enjoy and that you can stick with on a regular basis. Long-term consistency will produce the greatest benefits. Understand that this will NOT be an exercise program just to help you lose a few pounds and then you can stop. This will be a part of your diabetes therapy for as long as you have diabetes. You should consider it a regular and all-important ritual for your entire lifetime. You'll have to work other aspects of your life around your exercise program rather than just trying to fit it into your current habits wherever you can. It absolutely must be assigned one of the highest priorities in your life. If something in your schedule must be changed for special occasions, don't even consider omitting your exercise – ever – unless you're in the hospital and just can't move! Even then, do what exercise you can do. Use it or lose it!

Exercise to keep your bones and body strong. Exercise to give yourself more energy on a regular basis. Exercise to help control your weight. Exercise to feel and be healthier and happier. And, as a type II diabetic, exercise to help manage and control your blood sugar levels in a healthy, drug-free way.

Regeneration

So far, you've learned about several things that you need to do on a regular basis. It's also extremely important as a type II diabetic that you spend some time NOT doing things as well – in other words – getting some rest! Insufficient rest causes more stress. Additional stress from sleep loss and lack of enough rest is a major contributor to higher blood sugar levels.

But telling somebody to "get enough rest" is almost as tricky a piece of advice as telling somebody to "eat right and exercise." With all the different types of information out there, what in the world might "getting enough rest" actually mean?

Resting is certainly not an exact science. It varies from person to person. If you're a compulsively active person, for example, forcing yourself to stay in bed when you're chomping at the bit to get a lot of things done, could actually be providing you with more stress than it does true rest. Instead, you may want to just slow down some while still feeling productive.

The results of a late 1990's study on longevity and sleep were presented at an Activator Methods, Inc. seminar in Phoenix, Arizona, showing that for the average person, the optimum amount of sleep for a long, productive and healthy life is between seven and nine hours per night. According to this study, when the amount of average sleep was less than 7 hours or more than 9, maximum benefits and overall longevity decreased proportionately. I strongly recommend that type II diabetics aim for this optimum sleep range of 7 to 9 hours out of every 24.

However, when some people get less than 8 to 10 hours of sleep a night, they find it difficult to function to the best of their ability. According to historians, Winston Churchill, for instance, needed an average of 10 hours of sleep daily to function at his full potential.

A 2005 magazine article authored by one of the world's leading researchers on sleep and endurance athletes, like those who compete in endurance sailing, agrees. According to this expert, the maximum sleep benefit comes when you can get a regular six to nine hour nighttime sleep. But he also promotes the wonders of naps.

He says that from six to eight o'clock in the evening is the worst time to try to get a nap for a human being, citing evolutionary times in human development. This time frame was when nighttime predators were going out on the hunt and it was imperative to remain extra vigilant during this transition time from light to dark.

On the other hand, the best times for a nap are early to mid-afternoon and about three in the morning, traditionally the safest times to sleep in those historical times in terms of avoiding predators. Other times for naps may work out differently for individuals depending on their personal circumstances.

The author of that article suggested that the average person gets a minimum of six hours of sleep at night and then includes a fifteen-minute to half-an-hour nap in the mid afternoon. Considering all the above research, I personally recommend at least seven hours sleep with a mid day nap for the type II diabetic.

Recent articles have appeared in the corporate world about this concept of mid-day naps. You may have seen references to the new corporate "power nap" and how it's now making its way into mainstream American business. This is my personal favorite. I always try to get this short nap right after lunch, sitting in my "nap chair." When I get this little afternoon snooze in my office, I can perform at much higher levels with far less stress, more stamina, more accuracy and more endurance all the way through my very last patient of the day.

Sleep is a huge challenge for a the type II diabetic due to several common influences – pain, stress, restlessness, frequent nighttime urination (especially for diabetics), waking early and not being able to fall back asleep again, worries, emotional distress, fear, anger and the list goes on. Also of major consideration are heavy meals, poor food combining, caffeine use and both prescription and over the counter drugs.

As a chiropractor, of course, one of the most frequent causes of sleep loss that I see is chronic pain, a fairly easy symptom to address. This holds true whether the complaint is low back pain, neck pain, hip pain, knee pain, thumb pain or even jaw pain. It's an on-going cycle of stress creating increased blood sugar – high blood sugar increasing existing pain levels – pain causing on-going sleep loss and sleep loss causing more stress. An effective point at which to break this cycle is to address the pain in a natural way by eliminating its cause.

So if pain is a major influence that's keeping you awake, my very first recommendation would be to find a well-qualified chiropractor. An easy way to find a well-qualified one is to go on-line to www. activator.com, click on "certified doctors" and look for an "advanced proficiency rated" doctor of chiropractic near you. This may not be an infallible method of finding a good chiropractor, but it's a good place to start. It's a way to determine that the doctor has met at least a minimum standard of advanced, post-license training.

White willow bark is a natural anti-pain supplement as is Noni, a tropical fruit, both available at most health food stores. Anti-inflammatory foods include artichokes, asparagus, broccoli, cherries, cinnamon, and grapefruit. Typically, reducing inflammation reduces pain as well.

Some of the things I recommend to my patients when they still complain of sleep challenges after other avenues have fallen short include chamomile tea, valerian, either in capsule or tea form, lobelia (capsules), magnesium, passiflora (also known as passion fruit), vitamin C and Melatonin. I don't, however, recommend them all at once!

I usually start by recommending chamomile tea, half an hour before bedtime. There are also several sleep-helpful teas containing chamomile available at most grocery stores such as "Cozy Chamomile, Sweet Dreams" and "Sleepy Time" teas by Bigelow. If you don't care for the taste of chamomile tea, mix it half and half with your favorite DECAFF tea – Constant Comment or Bigelow Vanilla, for instance. I actually prefer the mixtures myself. If that's not enough to help you achieve adequate sleep, take three to six mg of Melatonin at the same time. (This combination alone knocks my lights out!)

If these aren't effective, I recommend replacing the chamomile tea with valerian either in tea form or in capsules. Valerian is a stronger sleep inducing herb than chamomile. If that doesn't do the trick, replace the valerian with the lobelia capsules (no more than three capsules though. It can nauseate you if you use too much). Lobelia is an even stronger sleep-inducing herb. It's calming effects have also been known to help people stop smoking!

I believe that anybody with sleep challenges, especially type II diabetics, should be sure to take about 500 mg to 1,000 mg of magnesium (magnesium citrate to be specific) and 4,000 mg of vitamin C daily, preferably in the evening.

Why so much vitamin C? Only three animals don't make their own vitamin C. Humans are one of those creatures. In the animal world, the ones who do make their own make an average of the equivalent of 4,000 mg per day when they're well and increase it to about 9,000 mg per day when they're sick. I use these numbers as a general guideline for human use of vitamin C and it seems to work well for myself, my family and my patients. It also coincides with, or perhaps is even a little less than, Linus Pauling's recommendations. He, as you may remember, won the coveted Nobel Prize for his research on vitamin C. This amazing supplement is particularly important for type II diabetics because of its specific healing properties.

Next, I recommend tryptophan as an amino acid that can help to promote sleep as well. It's difficult to find it as a separate supplement today in health food stores and it's somewhat expensive when you do. The best way to get plenty of tryptophan in amounts that help promote sleep, believe it or not, is to eat turkey. This is one of the reasons why twenty minutes to an hour after the typical Thanksgiving dinner, family members start passing out in front of the TV – tryptophan! It's also available as an ingredient in amino acid capsules or powders.

Why not use sleeping pills? The greatest danger in using sleeping pills is that they're drugs, whether they're the over-the-counter type or prescription medicines. They all have unwanted and undesirable side effects. Most often, the worst side effects are that they're addictive (manufacturers euphemistically call them "habit forming").

Another danger, although seldom mentioned, arises because they alter some very important aspects of the five stages of sleep that are each necessary for maximum health benefit. Drowsiness, light sleep, two stages of deep sleep and rapid eye movement (REM) sleep, the stage in which we dream, each serve specific purposes physically, emotionally and psychologically. Altering any one or all of them can have long-term detrimental effects. Just having your eyes closed and being unconscious doesn't necessarily mean that the sleep you're experiencing is accomplishing the same thing as natural, restorative sleep in all of its natural cycles.

In reference to Melatonin, this is a naturally occurring substance manufactured in your own brain in response to influence from the pineal gland. The pineal gland is believed to be the portion of the brain that's most sensitive to light other than the eyes themselves. In the absence of light, it produces Melatonin to induce sleep. In millennia past, this served a very good purpose for diurnal creatures – those that roamed during the day and slept at night. Today, when we're more concerned with clocks, schedules and appointments than with whether the sun is up or not, the process of Melatonin production, or the lack of it, is less important to us. We don't want to fall asleep at 7:00 or 8:00 PM, when the sun sets. We want to boogie till the wee hours of the morning or make extra money on the night shift!

We've lost our understanding of the importance of darkness, sacrificing it and its healing, sleep benefits for the feeling of security that light and seeing our surroundings can offer us. But in the process, we do pay the price.

So this is another, very important key to getting restful sleep. Make sure that your room is dark when you lie down for the night. It should be absolutely dark – pitch black. Even if you can't get it that dark, make it as dark as you can. If it's not dark where and when you're trying to sleep, you're sabotaging your efforts at slumber and your well being.

Stress is a major contributor to sleep loss too. Stress is medically defined as any stimulus that causes the secretion of cortico-steroids. Cortico-steroids are substances released by the adrenal cortex – substances like adrenaline and adrenaline-like steroids. Any pressure, fear, anger or anxiety we're experiencing puts us into what's known as a "fight or flight" state. When the adrenal cortex secretes its cortico-steroids, the pupils dilate, the blood is re-routed away from the skin and internal organs and toward the muscles. All body functions that don't contribute directly to either attacking an enemy or running away are shut down to their minimum activities. Muscle tension, hearing, vision and sensitivity to our surroundings heighten to prepare for lightning-quick actions and reactions in an instant – ready to either fight or flee. Just the opposite of what we want if sleep is our goal!

To reduce stress, there are some things to consider in your evening ritual activities before trying to go to sleep. As much as you can, avoid TV shows that get you really excited or disturbed just before bedtime. Things like watching the news, for instance, often work against our slumber attempts due to their affects on our adrenaline levels. Super-thriller action shows and scary horror shows that put us on the ends of our seats produce similar effects because they too put us into the fight or flight mode, even if passively. Give yourself a half an hour or so after these kinds of stimuli to relax and mellow out. Read something inspirational. Think about something calming. Meditate. Watch or read something funny. Do something that you think might help a person sleep with pleasant dreams rather than unpleasant ones. My wife, Linda, counts her blessings every night. It works well for her.

Why is sleep so important to the diabetic? When we're stressed (in the fight or flight state) our body is literally preparing to either engage in battle or run like mad. Either situation requires a sudden burst of energy. So in this state, the body calls on any energy stores it can, such as converting some fat into glucose, for immediately available energy. But then the diabetic can't get the glucose out of the blood and into the cells. In type I, it's because there isn't enough insulin, in type II, it's because the cells are resistant to even excessive amounts of insulin. Either way, the end result of stress is increased blood sugar, the most undesirable state for any diabetic. That increased blood sugar also contributes to frequent nighttime urination, another sleep robber. Conversely, you can minimize your overall stress levels by getting plenty of natural sleep.

Another way is to learn and practice relaxation techniques. Twenty minutes a day of sitting quietly, preferably with your eyes closed, without talking to anyone, listening to anyone or hearing conversations, no music with lyrics, no interruptions, no reading, just sitting alone, quietly, can work well for this. Soft, soothing, instrumental music is OK, however, if not recommended. Or try closing your eyes and singing the word HU. (Pronounced like "hue.") Sing it once with each long, drawn out breath, over and over, for about 20 minutes. An ancient, sacred name for God, it seems to have a calming and uplifting effect for most people. Sing it aloud when you're alone, or silently to yourself when others are around you.

The less you allow yourself to be upset by your surroundings, the less stress will develop, the less sleep loss will manifest, and the better you'll therefore be able to control your blood sugar in a natural way.

Establishing regular sleep patterns can also have a particularly beneficial effect for people who want to improve their sleep. Researchers state in study after study that people who practice a pattern of going to sleep and getting up at the same time every day have consistently better sleep than those who have no such patterns or frequently interrupted patterns. This can be a particular detriment for people whose work shifts change from week to week or month to month.

The bed you sleep in obviously affects your ability to sleep restfully too. Worn out mattresses and/or box springs are terrible culprits, responsible for inadequate rest. Sagging dips and holes in your mattress are clues that your bed could use replacing. They're evidence that your mattress can't support you at the crucial points and this allows your skeletal frame to distort while you're sleeping.

Pillows that raise your head too high or that are too flat can also cause sleep challenges by placing unnatural bends in your neck for hours at a time. Even as a chiropractor, I don't have much confidence in the chiropractic pillows. Memory foam or down-filled feather pillows earn my best recommendation. I've heard some good reports from people who've used the water pillows too.

Different people have different comfort levels in terms of mattress firmness. Some require soft mattresses, others firm ones. The ideal mattress for you is the one that allows you to sleep most soundly through the night with adequate support and which results in no pains or aches in the morning.

I'm not a great proponent of box springs for a bed either. I prefer a high-quality mattress on a firm platform. My own bed consists of a wood frame with a rigid plywood platform between the head board and the foot board. I bought the best mattress I could find and placed it directly on the solid wooden frame. The support is great and the mattress provides comfort for wonderful sleep.

When I decide to purchase a new bed in the future, after investigating many types of sleep systems, my first choice will be a Tempurpedic, the one with the space-age memory foam. The second choice would be a Sleep Number bed. I've used the Tempurpedic and have nothing but marvelous things to say about it, as do my patients who own them, even though it's a bit on the pricey side. But you get what you pay for.

Although I haven't had the occasion to actually experience a Sleep Number bed, I have patients who've bought them and have returned good reports. This bed also addresses the challenge of sleeping partners who have very different comfort levels when it comes to mattress firmness. Each side of this air-filled mattress can be adjusted to suit the individual.

Hopefully, this chapter has given you some insights into the importance of rest, how much is enough and how to adjust your rest periods to keep your sleep up to adequate levels. If you have sleep challenges, you now have some nutritional/supplemental resources to try and you have some considerations for making your sleep environment the most conducive to producing actual sleep. You also have some ways to change your pre-sleep time to prepare you better for sound, restful sleep.

Sleep / rest is when your body does the majority of its repair and has its greatest opportunity to re-balance its normal chemistry. Be certain to give it at least as high a priority as you do getting adequate amounts of exercise.

The Food Pyramids

After careful testing and research, I'm afraid I have no confidence in the traditional "Food Pyramid" that's been touted as the gold standard for diet over the past few decades. The Food Pyramid, if you're not familiar with it, encourages using carbohydrates – grains, fruits and vegetables as the mainstay for your diet and urges limiting proteins and restricting fats to a bare minimum.

The very first sign that this is not the most healthy way to go, especially if you're a type II diabetic, is that ever since the beginning of the Food Pyramid's promotion as the road map to healthy eating, America has gotten fatter and fatter, year after year, until today, America is more obese as a nation than it's ever been in history and suffering from all of the secondary ailments that are associated with it. And it's not getting any better, it's getting worse! The problem is so bad now that obesity in school children is at an all-time, epidemic high and a third of the population is significantly overweight!

Yet well-meaning dietitians continue to seek a convenient, if undeserving scapegoat, hoping to indict eating fat or eating in one category of restaurants as a single, "Big Culprit." Let's take a look at the reality, however.

You may have read about the following study. Not long ago a man who was generally healthy, with a healthy heart, circulatory system and healthy cholesterol levels decided to initiate a study of the king of fast food. For his research, he was to eat every meal for a month at McDonald's. He did, ordering everything he could order in "Super-size" and had his doctor document the results on an on-going basis during his research. His doctor begged him to terminate his scientific investigation before it was even complete however, because of the quickly increasing dangers to his heart, such as elevating cholesterol levels, blood pressure and his weight. Conclusion – eating at McDonald's is unhealthy, causes heart disease and makes you fat.

At about the same time, a woman decided to do another study by eating at McDonald's with similar parameters – every meal for 30 days was to be eaten at the Golden Arches. At the end of a full month, however, her cholesterol levels had gone down, her heart and arteries were fine and she had lost 20 pounds. Conclusion? Eating at McDonald's was a good and healthy eating plan.

How could this possibly be? Easy! It's a matter of understanding the foods available and taking responsibility for what we order and put into our mouths! This lady ordered in a responsible way, enjoyed some fatty foods but was conscious of the dangers of combining them with carbohydrates and she followed good food combining practices. Blaming America's weight problem on McDonald's or the general category of fast-food restaurants is simply an irresponsible red herring, a misguided attempt to shift the blame away from ourselves and our own choices and onto a convenient, catch-all fall guy. The problem with this kind of thinking is that discontinuing the feasts at McDonald's and Burger King won't change a thing if we don't learn what the real culprits are and then take full, personal responsibility for our own health!

Let's start with grains. The grains we eat today are nothing like the natural ones man first discovered and began to harvest for food. A great way to get some perspective on this is to pick up any box of easy-to-prepare rice from the store, then compare it to a bag of wild rice harvested from the wetlands by American Indians in Minnesota. The differences are obvious and huge. Even though they're certainly considered entirely separate species now and I have no evidence to back my hunch, I have to believe that our current, familiar, domestic rice started out in antiquity more similar to that Minnesota wild rice before it was developed as a farm crop thousands of years ago. At some point in history, before man began to plant and harvest grains, all rice was wild rice, by definition. We've made a lot of changes over the past few millennia, to the point that now the difference is dramatic.

Today, there are probably very few examples of ancient wheat except for the grains the archeologists have been able to rescue from the tombs of the ancient Egyptian pharaohs. Even then, wheat grain had already been "re-engineered" by selective breeding for centuries, if not millennia, to produce the most hardy strains that would yield the most abundant, large kernels and withstand long-term storage. Anytime a grain is bred for some sort of change of convenience for us, it undergoes other changes too that don't always work in our favor, even if we're not aware of it at the time.

Corn, another mainstay grain of the American diet, has been hybridized many, many times over the centuries to produce specialized strains, to make it less vulnerable to mechanical harvesting, shipping and marketing display. And despite all of the "benefits" we've been able to achieve with these deliberate changes, we've also changed some fundamental qualities we probably didn't want to change along the way or didn't even know that we were changing.

For instance, in my practice, I've been certified since 1998 to perform animal skeletal adjusting. Over the past few years, Tahya Aung Khin of Scottsdale, Arizona, has developed and marketed an amazing, grain-free food for dogs, called Real Animal Way (www. realanimalway.com). Similar foods have statistically reduced vet bills by an average of 73%. Ever since he first put it on the market, pet owners have reported that the pet food apparently minimizes or eliminates joint pains in their dogs. This phenomenon is so prevalent with customers that I now question every canine patient's owner about what they feed their dogs. The worst joint pain I see in the dogs is consistently when their owners feed them foods that are high in grain content, especially wheat and corn. Typically, when they change their dogs' foods to a grain-free diet, the joint pain reduces faster and more significantly than if I were doing skeletal adjusting alone.

So I've had the opportunity to see first-hand the destructive, painful effects that grains have on mammalian joints. Being mammals ourselves, and omnivores like dogs are, I must assume that these grains can have similar effects on our own joints.

When we take the dogs off of all dog foods containing grains, including rice, their arthritic joints get amazingly better – often to the extent that they need no further intervention in terms of skeletal adjusting. Their skin gets healthy, their fur gets shiny, their muscle mass increases, their body fat decreases and their breath freshens, just to name a few of the health benefits they enjoy. We've had great results with controlling blood sugar in diabetic dogs on this dog food too! I believe that grains have harmful effects on human joints, skin, hair and connective tissue as well, even if their effect may be less intense. And being high-carbohydrate foods, we know that they have detrimental effects on type II diabetes.

Therefore, the first objection I have to the grains and cereals portion of the traditional Food Pyramid is the effects they can have on our overall health. Being the sticklers Linda and I are for experimentation and noting results, we've worked with this theory to see how it affects our own health. Linda, for example, before she eliminated grains from her diet completely, discovered that she could stop eating wheat alone and drop 14 pounds in two weeks. Over a period of years, she did this several times with exactly the same result – 14 pounds in two weeks. (You might want to experiment with this yourself.)

Additionally, she had assumed for many years that eating meat caused her knees to become inflamed (arthritic). However, she eventually discovered that the most direct relationship between her knee pain and her diet was in relationship to eating grains, especially wheat, not meat at all! It seems then that the theory of dietary grains (especially wheat) causing joint inflammation is not only true for animals, but is also true in at least some humans.

How does this relate to diabetics? First, pain causes stress. Stress increases your blood sugar. Increased blood sugar is the cause of most of the symptoms and secondary ailments that diabetics experience. Secondly, grains, especially these three, (wheat corn and rice) are high in carbohydrates. Regardless of the fiber and/or protein they may contain, the bottom line for the type II diabetic is that they contain a lot of carbohydrates. So minimize their use or eliminate them entirely, if you can. They can only get you in trouble. Every food you'll ever eat will be turned into glucose, among other things, so you don't have to specifically depend on having any grains in your diet for any particular reason provided you are getting sufficient amounts of fiber from other sources (which is very easy).

The first category of foods at the broad base of the standard Food Pyramid (See figure I) is complex carbohydrates, pasta, grains and cereals. It includes breads and anything made from any type of flour, pie and quiche crusts, pastries, corn chips, corn meal, rice cakes, brown rice and all cereals. In direct contrast to the Food Pyramid originators, I believe that the less of these grains, pasta and carbohydrates you eat as a type II diabetic, the better off you'll be.

Pasta is usually made from wheat, buckwheat, corn or other grains, or a combination of one or more of these things and other ingredients like spinach. But wheat is a major ingredient in making most pasta. They may be categorized as "complex carbohydrates," but they are nonetheless carbohydrates and for most type II diabetics, will cause increased blood sugar levels.

Cereals are also grains. Even the most health-promoting cereals usually contain wheat, rice and/or corn in some form. These are, after all, the main cereal grains.

The Traditional Food Pyramid

("Poison" for the type II diabetic!)

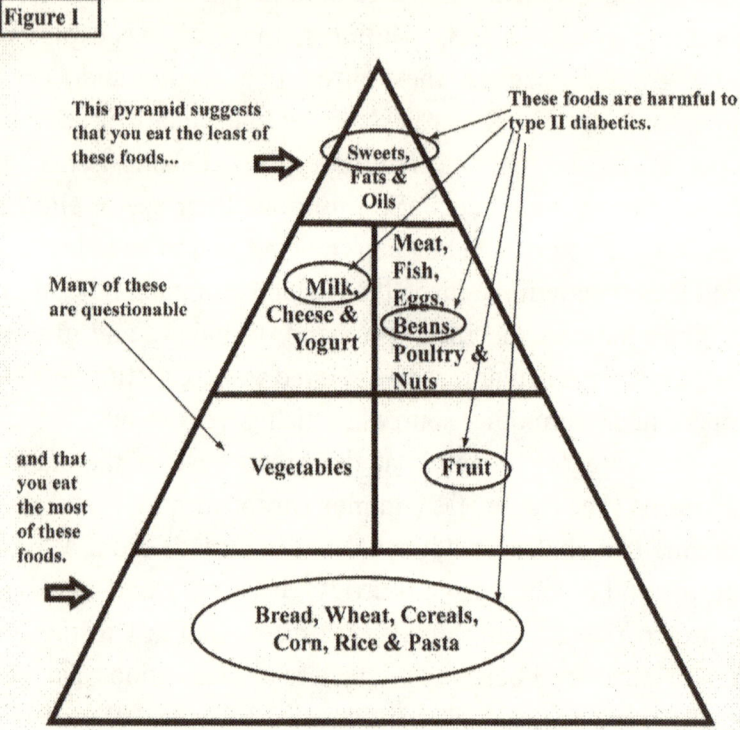

Figure 1

This pyramid suggests that you eat the least of these foods...

These foods are harmful to type II diabetics.

Sweets, Fats & Oils

Meat, Fish, Eggs, Beans, Poultry & Nuts

Many of these are questionable

Milk, Cheese & Yogurt

and that you eat the most of these foods.

Vegetables

Fruit

Bread, Wheat, Cereals, Corn, Rice & Pasta

Following this traditional Food Pyramid for the past thirty years has resulted in an average increase in the weight of Americans of 10 to 20 pounds. It can be a potent contributor to the development of type II diabetes and joint pains. Unfortunately, it also bears a striking resemblance to the Diabetic Food Pyramid created by the American Diabetic Association and the American Diabetes Association.   99A

Barley, millet, spelt and oats are also cereal grains. Like wheat, rice and corn, they contain significant proportions of carbohydrates. Although these are normally healthy grains for the non-diabetic, they should remain on the prohibited carbohydrate list for type II diabetics and avoided if you want to achieve maximum blood sugar control.

Some people argue that oatmeal, a grain, has been shown to reduce cholesterol in a natural way. True. But after what you've already learned about cholesterol in this book, you should understand the realities of cholesterol much better and have less fear of it. Next, please refer again to the chapter on cholesterol in this book and its connection to carbohydrates. Remember that the carbs in foods will cause the formation of serum cholesterol even more readily than eating high-cholesterol foods themselves. My recommendation for reducing cholesterol with diet, then, would be more to stay away from the carbs than to eat oatmeal that contains carbs if you're a type II diabetic. This may not hold true for those who don't suffer from diabetes or pre-diabetes, but is surely true for those who do.

Moving up the pyramid, it narrows, meaning that eating less of these foods is suggested. This next level up on the standard Food Pyramid is for fruits and vegetables. Again, I disagree with this category being recommended for diabetics with such a large portion of the diet consisting of high-carbohydrate fruits and high glycemic index vegetables. Let's look at how this part of the pyramid relates to the type II diabetic. Grains, pastas and the "complex carbohydrates" that are found in vegetables all introduce carbohydrates to our systems – poison for the type II diabetic. So, for diabetics, I believe that the current two levels at the base of the pyramid can and should be radically altered to minimize or eliminate as many carbohydrates as possible. This could prevent the huge and growing epidemic of type II diabetes in America and much of the obesity too!

Fruits are certainly wonderful foods and most people love them! They delight the Soul! However – when bought in the grocery store, you can be certain that they were picked prematurely, the beneficial enzymes did not have a chance to develop nor did the natural flavors. But unfortunately, they still contain great quantities of carbohydrates. Since all foods that we ever eat do introduce glucose into our systems – blood sugar, it's not actually necessary to consume carbohydrates in any particular form, not even in the form of fruits, especially when they seldom resemble real, tree-ripened fruit anyway.

I realize that it may be tough to give up fruits if you're diabetic, but understand that fruit, per se, is not a vital ingredient in itself to keep you healthy. If you must eat fruit, however, be very selective about it and strictly limit your consumption. For instance, eat a strawberry, maybe two, if your personal blood sugar reactions indicate that you can. But don't eat a whole bowl full. Don't eat frozen strawberries that have been prepared with sugar. Eat a fresh one. If you need to make them sweeter, add some stevia or Sweet & Low. You can even add a little cream if you like.

If you get a craving for citrus, buy a grapefruit. Peal it and divide it into sections. Eat one or two sections a day. No more. If you absolutely have to have an apple, buy one. Cut it into eighths or quarters and eat one part per day.

But stay completely away from the really high carb stuff like pineapples and bananas, especially fruits in dried form where the carbs are concentrated even more.

As a general rule, fruits should be extremely limited for the diabetic, especially those with type II. They should occupy only a tiny spot at the very top of your personal food pyramid – the area that indicates the least consumption of a food. (See illustrations.)

Vegetables, on the other hand, really should occupy a huge part of the pyramid at its base to achieve maximum health for the diabetic. This isn't to say that you should become a vegetarian. That's not at all necessary. But for the diabetic, vegetables should be the mainstay of the diet.

It's incredibly important to qualify this again, however. Some vegetables have high fiber content and very few carbs. There are other high-fiber vegetables with quite significant amounts of carbs that you must learn to avoid. Do your homework and learn the carbohydrate content of foods, then select those vegetables in the former category, those with little or no carbs at all. Limit the ones with medium carb content and eliminate those with high carbs.

Choose those with the fewest carbohydrates like broccoli, cabbage, lettuce, salad greens, spinach, radishes, cauliflower, zucchini, peppers, avocados and eggplant. Avoid veggies with high carb content including potatoes, sweet potatoes, carrots, and peas.

This is a very short list and there is a longer list at the back of this book, but you can, and should, pick up a carb-counter book at your local bookstore to look up and memorize your own favorites. The rule is that you should keep your carbohydrate intake to less than 30 grams per day if you're a type II diabetic. For some, it may even be less. Use your own testing supplies to determine what you can actually handle. The chapter on testing will give you more specifics on how to go about that.

You can eat veggies raw, as snacks or in salads. You can sauté them, fry them, grill them, broil, bake or even steam them. Enjoy them for all they're worth! They should make up the basis of your type II diabetic diet – the diet that can keep you off of the most drugs, and also keep you the most healthy.

The next level up on the traditional Food Pyramid, the next smaller level, suggests meats of all kinds, including beef, veal, pork, fish, other seafood, lamb and poultry. Also included are nuts, eggs, milk and milk products like yogurt, and cheeses.

For type II diabetics, I agree that this category level should be atop the vegetables, that you should consume less from this category than vegetables, but you should absolutely eat more foods from this category than from the fruits, cereals and grains categories. We discussed what adequate amounts of protein are in the chapter on protein. But just to refresh your memory, it's 1.5 grams of protein for every pound of body weight per day. There are 28 grams in a ounce. Meats are proteins. Nuts have significant amounts of proteins too, but use caution here. Some nuts are rather high in carbs, such as cashews. Others are more forgiving, such as almonds and walnuts. All contain some carbs so eat them sparingly and test to see what your own body can handle.

The top of the current traditional Food Pyramid is sweets and desserts. I agree that this should be the category of foods consumed the least, whoever you are. But it doesn't have to be eliminated for the diabetic if you make a few healthy changes.

Linda is one of the most sensitive people I know to any kind of carbohydrate. A few pecans will spike her blood sugar, as will a single strawberry sometimes. However, she has created some delicious desserts for us that even she can eat from time to time.

With an inexpensive home ice cream maker, she makes home-made ice cream using heavy cream, NOT MILK or half and half. She uses stevia and small amounts of Sweet & Low, sometimes adding sugar-free Jell-O to give it a smoother texture and fruit flavor. She's made it with coffee and/or Torani sugar-free syrups for other flavors like chocolate, vanilla or caramel.

She makes a great crust-less cheesecake using walnut crumbs where the crust would be. She makes a fantastic trifle using baked meringues in place of lady fingers, custard in place of pudding, real whipped cream sweetened with stevia and/or Sweet & Low, and a few slices of a strawberry for accent.

She makes meringue cookies with various ingredients using different techniques to achieve various textures from super-light and crispy to nearly a brownie texture. You don't have to give up the desserts. You only have to be creative and eliminate the parts of them that are poison to the type II diabetic.

Following the current traditional Food Pyramid for the diabetic is a treacherous journey that leads to certain degeneration of the type II diabetic condition. I say this in no uncertain terms. I believe that it's not only unsafe for type II diabetics to follow this traditional Food Pyramid, but that it's actually one of the most potent contributors to obesity and the development of type II diabetes in all of America.

So I've developed what I call the Diabetic Survival Pyramid (DSP). (See figure II) I want to point out specifically that the DSP is very different from the "Diabetic Food Pyramid" published by the American Diabetes Association and the American Diabetic Association which bears an amazing resemblance to the traditional Food Pyramid.

The Diabetic Survival Pyramid

(For Maximum Health and Longevity!)

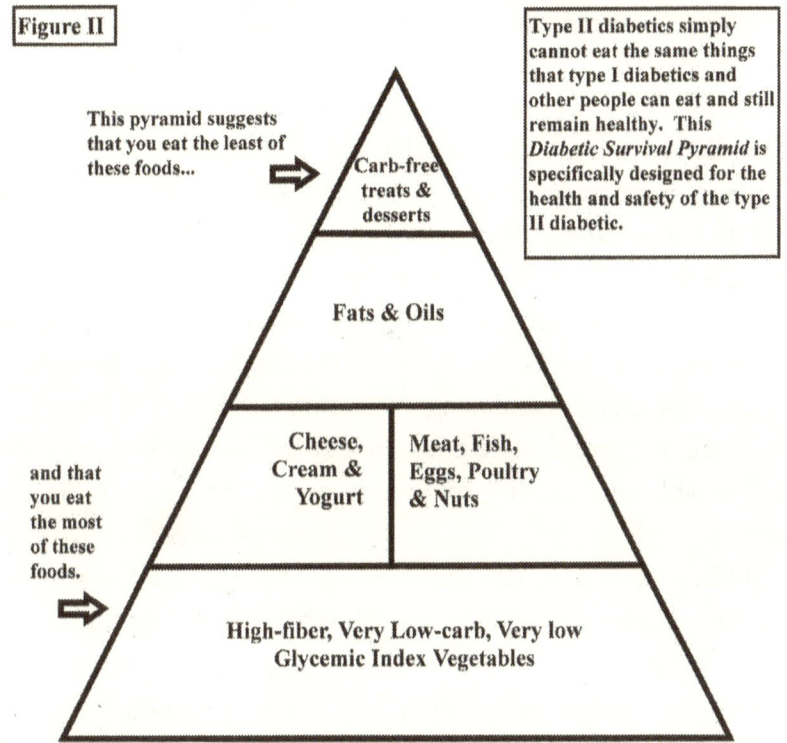

Figure II

This pyramid suggests that you eat the least of these foods...

Carb-free treats & desserts

Type II diabetics simply cannot eat the same things that type I diabetics and other people can eat and still remain healthy. This *Diabetic Survival Pyramid* is specifically designed for the health and safety of the type II diabetic.

Fats & Oils

Cheese, Cream & Yogurt

Meat, Fish, Eggs, Poultry & Nuts

and that you eat the most of these foods.

High-fiber, Very Low-carb, Very low Glycemic Index Vegetables

Note that some of the foods on the traditional Food Pyramid aren't even listed on the *Diabetic Survival Pyramid*. You should either eliminate or minimize their use! These foods include bread and other baked goods, wheat, cereals, corn, rice, pasta, most fruits, potatoes, high glycemic index vegetables and sugar in any form.

99B

At the bottom of the DSP, the base of the pyramid that I recommend you follow, is vegetables with an extremely low carbohydrate content and a high fiber content. This should be the majority of the type II diabetic's diet. A small portion of these vegetables can contain limited amounts of carbohydrates but should never be enough to cause the diabetic to actually excrete sugar in the urine. This tolerable carbohydrate amount will vary from person to person. High-carbohydrate vegetables should be avoided, period.

The next level up on the DSP is proteins, fats and dairy products. This includes 1.5 grams of protein per pound of body weight daily. This category can include sugar-free yogurt, many cheeses (depending on how they affect your blood sugar), heavy cream in your coffee or tea (but do not use powdered creamer or milk). Half and half is OK but not the greatest. Cream is what you want to use.

Use butter, not margarine. Margarine is dangerous. It's far more likely to cause cancer than butter! Margarine is made from long-chain unsaturated oils which are vulnerable to heat in the extraction process. In the curriculum presented when I took my nutrition studies in college were warnings about the unpredictable breakdowns of these long-chain oils during extraction. Evidence suggests that they break at unpredictable points under heat and pressure creating unpredictable molecules - some toxic, even carcinogenic (cancer-causing).

Studies in *"The Cholesterol Myth"* by Sheldon Zerden, cite margarine as more dangerous than butter for the same reason.

The biggest caution that I could possibly give you in this category of foods is to refrain from eating fatty foods IN COMBINATION WITH CARBOHYDRATES! The fats without the carbs can be quite beneficial. Combine them with carbs and you create triglycerides, one of the truest threats to cardiovascular well-being.

The healthiest choices for vegetable oils, especially cooking oils, are olive oil (especially extra-virgin or cold-pressed), nut oils, coconut oil and avocado oil. They are more resistant to producing free radicals.

Eat fried eggs and bacon or a steak for breakfast with cream in your coffee, for instance, but if you include toast or potatoes, you're flirting with real danger. Have a fat, juicy cheeseburger for lunch with lettuce, pickles, mustard and mayonnaise. Even make it a double if you like! But leave the bun, the tomato and French fries on the plate and pass on the catsup to avoid mixing the fats and carbs.

At the top of the DSP are sweets and desserts, just as in the traditional pyramid, but with the exception that no sugar is allowed, even here. Refer to the chapter on When You Just Have To Have Something Sweet. Note that grains and cereals are not included in the DSP at all. For type II diabetics, they're poison. Fruits are not included as a category either. Keep them to a bare minimum. They should be just a speck at the very top of the DSP Food Pyramid. You can get all the nutrition you need from other sources that will help you more than fruits. No beans are allowed in the DSP either because of their high carbohydrate content.

This DSP pyramid is based on research demonstrating what works for controlling blood sugar, the most important single activity for physical and psychological survival in diabetics. It's simply impossible to eat like non-diabetics (or even like type I diabetics) and maintain your best possible levels of health. Uncontrolled blood sugar brings severe symptoms such as depression, anger, loss of feeling, loss of limbs, heart attacks and death to diabetics. This simple tool, the DSP, can help you to control that most deadly of all foes to the diabetic – your abnormal metabolism of blood sugar.

Don't let a pyramid be a tomb for you. Throw that old one out. Forget about it. It's poison for the type II diabetic! In my own estimation, the Diabetic Food Pyramid created by the American Diabetic Association and American Diabetes Association is just as dangerous! Instead make some healthy changes. Get a new road map. Adopt the Diabetic Survival Pyramid.

Testing

Linda and I are left nearly speechless with the commercials on TV when people announce, "I'm diabetic and I test 10 times a day!" We look at each other with our mouths hanging wide open and say, in unison, "Why?!" There's no therapeutic value in that at all! In fact, one of the dangers that both types of diabetics face is a reduced ability to heal in the extremities. So logic alone tells us that puncturing the fingers (or the forearm) that many times a day actually increases the risks of complications, the possibility of infections and in extreme cases, ultimately, the loss of limbs. So we'll be discussing testing procedures in this chapter and making suggestions for what I consider to be reasonable frequencies.

There are two categories of testing in this chapter – urine stick testing and meter testing. The urine sticks test for both the presence and amount of sugar in the urine and for the presence and amount of ketones. One type of urine testing sticks is called "Diastix." Diastix test for sugar in the urine only. "Ketostix," another type of urine testing sticks test for ketones in the urine only. "Ketodiastix," another type of testing sticks, have two pads on each stick so you can test for both sugar and ketones at the same time.

Walgreens has a store brand of these testing strips that are much less expensive and just as accurate.

The second type of testing is testing your blood with a glucose meter. There are several brands of testing meters available. They vary in size and ease of use. Some require a larger drop of blood than others.

All meters require you to present a drop of blood for testing. In order to remain safe and prevent infections and contamination, the "lances" you'll use with your meter for getting your drops of blood will be one-time-use lances. You'll need to buy them by the box. You'll also need to supply your meter with testing strips for each individual test. So it will also be necessary to buy these by the box. The use of different meters involves different pain levels too, depending on how much blood each meter requires in order to give you an adequate reading.

The cost of these supplies varies substantially from meter system to meter system.

Feel free to discuss your needs with your pharmacist regarding the price of the meters, the ease and price of replenishing your meter supplies, the ease of use of different meters and the comfort levels of using each meter.

These meters test for blood sugar levels. The ideal twelve-hour fasting blood sugar range is from 70 to 120 mg/dl. A range of from 120 to 180 mg/dl is considered by many to be a "borderline" range. Above 180, most doctors would give a diagnosis of diabetes. If your blood sugar is between 120 and 180 and there's no sugar in the urine, however, you may well be pre-diabetic. That is to say that your blood sugar is being held in check (even if ineffectively) only by massively over-active insulin responses. For diabetics, the most frequent challenge, of course, is blood sugar levels that are too high.

In terms of actual definitions, diabetes means the presence of sugar in the urine. So regardless of the actual meter reading of the blood sugar, if there's no spilling of sugar into the urine, it's not actually diabetes in the truest sense of the definition. It's only hyperglycemia – hyper meaning "too much" and glycemia meaning "sugar in the blood."

This can make a difference in how you'll want to test. The first thing you'll need to accomplish as a diabetic is getting your daily blood sugar down to a level that keeps your body from needing to get rid of sugar through the urine.

The way to do this is to test for sugar in the urine using your Diastix and adjust your daily intake of carbohydrates downward until your urine Diastix readings are consistently at zero. Actually, until you reach this first goal, there's little value in also using a meter to test your blood sugar unless you just want to know what the actual numbers are. If you're spilling sugar into your urine, there's simply too much blood sugar, period, so there's no need to risk puncturing your skin to measure it. You know you have to reduce your carbohydrate intake more.

Regardless of any theoretic numbers at which, or below which, anyone recommends that you keep your carbohydrate intake, your own, personal testing procedures will be the only VALID indicator of what will actually be true for you, individually. Everybody is different. You may be able to tolerate a little more, or you may not tolerate as much as those recommendations indicate in theory.

So, first use your Diastix to monitor the sugar in your urine. It's up to you as to how often to check it but do check it at least daily. In the beginning, it's helpful to get at least a morning fasting reading before you eat breakfast and another somewhere between 4 and 6 P.M. You may also want to test a few times during the day. An hour or two after meals, will be sufficient. Once you've learned how to keep the sugar in your urine at zero by eating various foods and then testing the results with your Diastix, you can then probably reduce the use of the Diastix to once daily, preferably before breakfast.

When you've achieved the point of keeping the sugar in your urine to zero, you can begin to fine tune your food repertoire by using your glucose meter. With the meter, you may want to take readings about three to four times daily, first on arising then about two hours after meals. I believe that testing more often than this is overkill and any value it might have would be overshadowed by the extra risks to your health that frequently puncturing the skin in your extremities presents.

Your first goal with the meter is to get your fasting blood sugar down to 180 or less, keeping in mind that this is only the borderline level. Again, eat foods and test for the results of those foods on your blood sugar with your meter. Adjust your daily carbohydrate intake until you've achieved the goal of 180. Once you've achieved this point, the ultimate goal is to reduce it to 120 or less. Work with it patiently! You don't have to accomplish this in a single month or even in a single year and many diabetics will require a few years to reach this level, even with consistent discipline. But be diligent and persistent. Make changes but make them gradually enough for them to become PERMANENT changes. After testing regularly for a few months, however, most people will be able to recognize some basic patterns and can reduce the testing frequency to once or twice daily.

It may take one, two or even several years to get the blood sugar down to these ideal levels by an all natural means, and it may require more than just changing the things you eat and drink and the supplements that you use. Exercise plays a vital part in the process, as you read in the chapter on exercise. You can bet, however, that whatever you do, it will take more than a few weeks or even a few months. It took years for your body to develop type II diabetes. It will take years to make significant changes in the way your body works, taking it back in the other direction.

Realistically, your choices are to work with it naturally and patiently to re-establish your health and well-being, or to take prescription drugs which only deal with the *symptoms* and in the mean-time allow the *real* problem(s) to get worse and worse over the years.

In this book, the goal is to bring your type II diabetes under control naturally. We know that drugs are dangerous and always present risks. That's why they're available by prescription only! And we know that absolutely all drugs have side effects. In the case of Glucophage, ("gluco-" referring to glucose, AKA blood sugar, and "phage" meaning "eater") the drug may reduce blood sugar by "gobbling up" or destroying glucose in the blood stream, but there's no way it can limit itself to just the glucose that's created by eating carbohydrates. It must also gobble up the glucose produced from eating fats and the glucose produced from eating proteins as well. Consequently, your body can be starving even though you're eating well or even over-eating. Also, Glucophage seems to be unable to prevent carbohydrates from binding with fats to become triglycerides ("heart poison") or to prevent the carbohydrates from contributing to increased body fat accumulation.

N. B. for instance was diagnosed in the late 1990's with type II diabetes. His weight of well over 300 pounds was a lot, even for his very large frame. A very active man who worked outdoors, one would expect that he would be able to keep an adequate check on his weight from the hours he spent in the field, walking.

His doctors at the Veterans Administration recommended a dietary program similar to the American Diabetes Association's Diabetes Food Pyramid described in the previous chapter and he was diligent about keeping the portions down. They also prescribed Glucophage which he takes regularly as prescribed.

Over the ensuing years, his weight has steadily increased, he has suffered from long bouts of depression and is often intolerant of people in his surroundings. I respect his right to choose the course of action he follows to manage his type II diabetes; however, his case illustrates some of the shortcomings of taking Glucophage and the following Diabetic Food Pyramid as a treatment paradigm.

Artificially reducing measurements of the blood sugar level alone, with drugs, therefore doesn't appear to address the entire picture by a long shot, but rather seems to create an illusion that leaves us with a false sense of well-being. In my patients who suffer from diabetes and take Glucophage, the typical health complications of the disease still manifest abundantly, even though the blood sugar levels may be somewhat lower on their meter readings. Actually, in many cases, because these patients feel a false sense of security, thinking that the drugs are really "controlling" the diabetes, they feel as though they can take liberties to indulge in foods that challenge their blood sugar and further compromise their health. Consequently, even though they take these strong, dangerous, prescription medications, there's little or no difference in the blood sugar levels of these people who are on drugs and those who work at it from a purely natural approach. I can only wonder why anybody would take dangerous prescription drugs if there's so little actual benefit, especially when they're so incredibly expensive!

I've seen at least one individual reduce blood sugar readings from 480+ to under 180 within 12 months using the strictly natural approaches described in this book. I've seen people whose blood sugar levels were over 300 submit themselves to using Glucophage and still have difficulty keeping their blood sugar levels under 250, either because no one has explained the dietary aspects of type II diabetes to them or they just didn't want to admit that they needed to change their diet to keep their blood sugar under control. The cold, hard truth is that there's actually no short cut around a controlled diet!

You can learn to consider your testing procedures as your friends and allies in your quest to live a long, comfortable, healthy life. They're like the steering wheel in your car. They're simply tools to help you come back to center, to stay on the right track from one day to the next. When you stray off course, they help you to recognize that and to steer back to the center. And, like using any kind of steering device, once you've established your objective, it takes much less effort to stay on course than it did to get you there originally. So once you've discovered the foods that lead you astray, by using your procedures of eating and follow-up testing, you can identify and eliminate those harmful foods. Then you can reduce the amount of testing you do on a daily basis because you'll already know how the foods that you like to eat affect you.

If you suffer from type II diabetes already and don't have the appropriate testing supplies at home, go out *today* and get them for yourself. There's no prescription necessary to buy these testing supplies, so there should be no excuses for you not to get them.

If you have challenges with constant hunger, climbing weight and think that there may be a possibility that you may be either pre-diabetic or type II diabetic, get some testing supplies right away and begin using them. Get some numbers. Do some experimenting so that you can gain control of your life, your health, your moods and your comfort levels. Information for the masses is always, by definition, generalized information. Your own individual parameters are specific numbers that you must find for yourself. The only way to accomplish that is by testing.

There are scores of books about diabetes written by all sorts of people with nutritional credentials and medical credentials urging you to eat the "good carbs" and avoid the "bad carbs" if you're diabetic. I contend that any of them that tout the use of any kind of carbs simply do not understand the difference between type II and type I diabetes. If you're type I and using insulin, go for it. If you're type II, I have serious doubts backed by all of the information you've read in this book so far. You can, and should, prove or disprove it to yourself, however. I don't think you should even take my opinion at face value. Buy your testing supplies. Test yourself with every kind of food the experts say for you to eat. Sometimes they may be right. Too often for us, they've been very wrong! The numbers you get from *your own* testing procedures will tell you what's true for you, individually.

There are also some helpful medical tests you won't be able to do for yourself but can have a doctor order for you. These tests usually only need to be done once or twice a year (if that often). They include:

1) a "free" and "bound" insulin test
2) an A1C test
3) a two-hour "post-prandial" glucose test and
4) a 12 hour fasting glucose test

Your doctor will know what these specific insulin tests are and what they're for.

Be sure that you get to see what the resulting numbers of the tests are and what the normal values should be. The first test is to determine your actual insulin levels. Higher than normal levels are of the greatest concern. Even if 12 hour fasting glucose levels are normal, accompanying high insulin levels suggest a pre-diabetic or type II diabetic condition.

I would never have a glucose tolerance test myself, however, nor would I ever recommend one for my patients. I believe that this test is too dangerous for a type II diabetic or a pre-diabetic. Such a large and concentrated dose of pure glucose has the potential to hospitalize many of them if they are, in fact, type II diabetics, or may even push a pre-diabetic into true diabetes, according to many healthcare professionals.

This battery of tests, without the glucose tolerance test, will give you a more reliable picture of what's happening with both your blood sugar and its relationship to your insulin, and thus, a better understanding of the status of your carbohydrate metabolism.

When You're Away From Home

Planning our meals and snacks and staying disciplined at it are a lot more simple to do when we're at home. We just buy the right things at the grocery store so that we always at least have the opportunity to make the correct choices and avoid temptations. If you're single, or you live with someone who feels comfortable following a similar eating plan, that makes it easier too. For instance, my wife has type II diabetes and I'm at least pre-diabetic. So we follow a very similar approach. It makes it easier for us both.

It's a far bigger challenge when you're at someone else's home, at a restaurant or you're on a trip and want to have a snack. The primary consideration here is to have a pre-determined strategy so that you remain in control. I simply cannot overstate the importance of having this pre-determined strategy. Without it you'll be subject to too many temptations, too many variables and too many opportunities to get yourself into trouble nutritionally.

Let's start with the easiest of these scenarios to control, snacks. Linda and I like to travel as do many Americans. One of the things that became incredibly apparent soon after she developed her diabetes was how very high in carbs virtually all commercially marketed snack foods are. Even the snacks that are labeled as low "net carbs" are almost always high in total carbohydrates and profoundly affect blood sugar levels for many type II diabetics. So leaving home trusting that you'll be able to find convenient snacks in your travels is usually a naïve assumption that will usually get you in trouble.

The best way to maintain control and still be able to have snacks when you travel is to prepare your own snacks before you leave home. But be sure to take some of the things you like, perhaps some meringue cookies (see the chapter on When You Just Have to Have Something Sweet), or some cubes of your favorite cheese. We like to take smoked salmon and cream cheese, some walnuts or smoked almonds, some slices of prosciutto-cheese rolls or some ham chunks.

When you're preparing your snacks, consider how long you're going to be between grocery store visits where you'll be able to take the time to shop. Buy a cold-pack of some kind to keep in your snack bag so you can keep cheeses and meats cool and prevent spoilage.

We always prepare this kind of a snack bag when we know we're going to be on the road for several hours. Since we know that it's just a good health practice for the spine to stop and stretch at least every hour when we're driving, this makes it really convenient to stop, stretch our legs and enjoy the snacks in a way that we know won't create a mess inside the car. After doing this for the past few years, we actually find our trips more enjoyable than they used to be when we just grabbed commercially packaged snack foods and sodas on the run.

In the airport, it's also very difficult to find carb-free snack foods or meals. So we bring a snack bag when we fly too. We can enjoy foods we love while waiting to board, and once we're on the plane, we're not spending $10 or more on a small sandwich and cookies, which are basically poison to diabetics anyway. And there's the added benefit that we're eating foods that we've personally chosen. We've found that by eating our own, carb-free or very low carb snack foods instead of airport and airline fare, we have much less jet lag and we don't pack on the pounds like we would if we had to rely solely on what they offered, not to mention that we feel much better during and after our vacations!

Restaurant eating is the next challenge. Eating at a restaurant is an activity that's unavoidable when we're traveling and from time to time, we just don't want to cook at home. We want somebody else to cook and do the dishes, or we want to just enjoy some of the great and unique foods that certain restaurants have to offer. When some people start restricting their carbohydrates, they're only sure of a few things they can eat, but that can get really boring, really fast! The trick to sticking with it, basically saving your life, is to become truly aware of the variety that you can have so that you can still fully enjoy the culinary arts.

Here are a few basic guidelines that can get you some tasty delights in nearly any kind of a restaurant. It just takes a little discipline and practice.

Since my wife and I are from Arizona and simply love Mexican food, let's start there. When they bring the chips and salsa, be aware that each chip has about a gram of carbohydrates. If you're keeping your carbs below 20 or 30 for an entire day, it doesn't take long for these to add up. In addition, there are tomatoes with carbs in the salsa. It's very easy to sit and talk while chomping down the chips and salsa unconsciously. *Don't!* If you're going to indulge, decide *beforehand* how many chips you'll eat and *stop* at that number. Ideally, pass on the chips and save the salsa to enjoy on your entre.

Steak picado is a good choice as is carne asada. Both are basically meat without many carbs in the preparation. Some of the restaurants offer chorizo and eggs, almost all protein. Seafood, chicken or beef burros or chimichangas offer a great taste with few carbs as well; however, if you must restrict your carbs severely, you may want to eat the stuffing out of the burros and chimichangas and leave the tortilla on your plate. The same is true of beef, chicken or fish tacos. The insides are great. The tortillas are questionable. Always ask your waiter or waitress to hold the rice and beans since both are very high in carbs and should be avoided by type II diabetics (see the Diabetic Survival Pyramid).

As the sauces go, where there are sauces, there are usually carbohydrates. Indulge in them very sparingly. But feel free to glob on the guacamole and sour cream.

In general, limit tomatoes, sauces and tortillas. Have fun with the meat, seafood, chicken and veggies. Pass on the desserts and alcohol. Iced tea always goes really well with Mexican food. Avoid drinking milk!

Steak houses can be high on the list for the type II diabetic. Most offer a great salad bar. But pass on the puddings, regular Jell-O, pasta and potato salads. Avoid the diet salad dressings. They're usually low fat but rich in carbs (not to mention that they taste weird!). Choose blue cheese, vinegar and oil or Ranch.

The home-made bread served hot and smelling wonderful should only be enjoyed with the nose. *Don't eat it!* If you just can't resist, ask the waitress to take it away or not to bring it in the first place.

Order whatever kind of meat you want from the grill but avoid breaded meats. The only consideration is how much it takes to satisfy you. But avoid the A-1 and other kinds of steak sauces because they typically contain lots of sugar(s).

If you have a yen for dessert, try coffee or decaff with lots of cream, sweetened with stevia or Sweet & Low to taste and consider that as dessert.

We were disappointed when we finally realized how forbidding Chinese food was for most type II diabetics. Even though it's rich with great vegetables and sparing on the meat, we've never found a sauce served in a Chinese restaurant that wasn't high in carbs and every dish has sauces with hidden sugars. The meats are also coated with either sauces or breading – high carb content additions. And to top it off, most Chinese food is served with rice, a high-carb food that's also often a joint-pain-producing grain. But if you find yourself out-voted in a crowd that insists on a Chinese restaurant, keep to the meat and/or vegetable dishes and avoid the rice. Have pot stickers but eat the insides and leave the outer dumpling. Eliminate as much of the sauce as you can from your order and either avoid the breaded meats or remove the breading.

It may seem to be a lot of extra work and a lot of discipline to muster; however, you'll really be glad you did. You'll feel much better because you'll be controlling your blood sugar much more effectively. The rewards will include fewer headaches, fewer bouts of indigestion or reflux, less energy drain, fewer infections and fewer feelings of crabbiness, not to mention you won't be hungry an hour later!

Italian food presents some challenges as well but they can be overcome in the better Italian restaurants. The biggest no-no, of course, is pasta, the backbone of Italian cuisine. That still leaves things like meatballs, seafood, veal and fish.

Another big challenge in the Italian restaurant is the garlic bread. It smells so wonderful and tastes so good! But limit your enjoyment of the garlic bread to smelling it. That way you'll be able to keep from having to pay for it with your health and well-being later on. Ask the waiter or waitress to take it back to the kitchen if you tend to give in to temptation.

Coffee with cream and non-sugar sweetener also make for a nice dessert replacement after a great Italian dinner. Avoid the spumoni and tiramasu!

Just a short word about pizza – eat all the toppings you like but leave the crust and don't order pineapple as one of the toppings. The tomato sauce is a gray area. It will depend on how well your own body handles it. Eat and test to determine your personal parameters.

Hamburger joints are America's favorite, despite how badly people talk about them. Serving food quickly is not a bad thing even though the "experts" harp on the evils of "fast food." It all comes down to taking responsibility for what you order and, ultimately, put into your body.

Feel free to get the biggest, juiciest double or triple burger you want. But when it comes, be absolutely sure you remove the bun! For instance a Burger King Double Whopper with cheese has 54 grams of carbohydrates, enough to make a conscientious type II diabetic shudder! But remove the bun and it only has 4 grams – an incredible difference! Those 4 grams probably come from the catsup and the tomato. Eliminate them too ("have it your way") and it can be at or near zero!

Avoid the fries as if they were edible plague! Shakes are a double whammy – sugar plus homogenized milk. Salads are tricky at the fast food places. The salads themselves are usually very good, or at least okay. But the trimmings and dressings are where the challenging, sneaky obstacles come into play. Croutons are bread, a major no-no for diabetics. So pass on the croutons. Be cautious about putting chili on your salad like they offer at Wendy's because it contains high-carb beans and tomato sauce. And before you assume you're doing well by just eating a salad, *read the label* on the salad dressing you'd pour on top of it. As often as not, even the ranch-style dressings at the fast food restaurants have high carbohydrate contents. I've seen them as high as 13 grams in a single packet (about two tablespoons)! It might be a good idea to have your own dressing with you when you order salads at the fast food place.

If a single hamburger just isn't enough for you without the bun, get two, but leave the carbs – the buns, side orders and desserts – alone. You'll be amazed at how well you can feel even though you're eating fast food. The fat's not very harmful if you don't have the carbs along with it.

The same goes for places like Arby's and Subway. Eat the roast beef, or the sandwich innards but throw away the bread. We usually take the bread home and give it to the blue jays in our yard! Be very aware that the sauces contain lots of carbs.

If you're craving fried chicken, go for it, but peel off the breaded skin. The skin itself isn't a problem, but the breading on it certainly is. Colonel Sanders now offers roasted, skinless chicken filets too that are pretty tasty. Cole slaw is all right if it has no sugar in it, but no biscuits, no corn, no mashed potatoes or gravy. Also avoid the pot pies. As delicious as they might be, not even counting the crust, they have a lot of flour (wheat) in them and high-carb veggies like peas and carrots.

Vietnamese and Thai restaurants can offer really flavorful delights. But, again, be aware of sauces and soups that have thickeners and avoid rice and anything breaded. Some Thai dishes also contain potatoes. *Don't eat them!* And if you order one of those wonderfully delicious Chai drinks, make certain it's sugarless. If it's not – pass on it.

Going out for breakfast is one of life's great joys. You can savor a great breakfast out if you'll observe just a few guidelines. For the majority of Americans, breakfast is probably the highest carbohydrate content meal they eat. But it certainly doesn't have to be. First, forget the juice. It's really high in carbs, even if it's just V8. Juice, in fact, is more or less a concentrated form of fruits (or vegetables). If you absolutely have to have some kind of juice, order water with a single wedge of lemon. Squeeze the lemon slice into your water. If you like, add a little carb-free sweetener.

Second, avoid everything on the menu that contains wheat (flour). This includes toast (even whole wheat toast), biscuits, gravy, muffins, English muffins, bagels or rolls of any kind. Just consider them to be the poison that they truly represent for all type II diabetics.

Third, most restaurants want to serve you some kind of potatoes, (or grits in the deep South) with your breakfast. Either ask them to hold these starchy little treats or consider them mere decorations on your plate. They are not for you to consume! Give them to someone else in your party if you like, but don't eat them yourself.

Pancakes are about the most dangerous food you could possibly order for breakfast. They're diabetic suicide! They're high-carb, flour cakes on which you add butter and either pour syrup (liquid sugar) or jelly or jam (fruit-flavored sugar).

What can you have? All the eggs you want – fried, scrambled, in an omelet, poached, soft boiled, hard boiled – whatever. But eggs can be pretty boring by themselves, right? So have some bacon, sausage, ham, steak, Canadian bacon or whatever kind of meat you'd like to have with them. If you have an omelet, add some cheese, mushrooms, onions, peppers, chilies and/or meat. You can even throw a tablespoon of sour cream on top. It's yummy! If you can handle tomatoes, try a little salsa on your eggs or your omelet.

Have some coffee with rich, heavy cream. Or splurge and have a breve – a café latte made with half and half or cream instead of milk. If your fancy coffee vendor has sugar-free syrups, try a mocha or a Milky Way mocha (chocolate and caramel syrups added). You can usually even indulge in a dollop of whipped cream on top since it's mostly air anyway.

Having protein for breakfast is a good idea in any case because it breaks down slowly and provides you with continuous energy throughout the first half of the day without the mid-morning slump your co-workers often feel after eating their high-carb breakfasts or no breakfast at all.

You can find such breakfasts just about anywhere, including some airports! In fact, this is about the easiest meal to do well with when you're traveling. You can even find them at McDonald's. If you order the McDonald's breakfast sandwiches, just remove the bread or the biscuit. If one's not enough without the bread, order two or three and throw the bread away!

If you want to go somewhere for a breakfast burrito, ask them to hold the potatoes and consider that there will be a handful of carbs in the tortilla and make allowances for it in your daily carb count.

Seafood restaurants can be a real treat. But there are yummy things you'll want to say no to as well. For instance, Red Lobster serves some great tasting cheese biscuits while you're waiting for your meal. Please, don't even take the cover off the basket! They'll get you in trouble. Just drink your tea and talk instead.

It's best to avoid seafood with breading on it such as deep fried shrimp, clams and scallops. But if you can get the breading off, go for it. These foods are usually offered prepared in alternative ways that are delicious too – sautéed in butter, in garlic sauce, shrimp cocktails, etc. Lobster is yummy and feel free to dip each luscious bite in the hot lemon butter. The fat's not really a problem in the absence of carbohydrates. Order an all-you-can-eat plate of anything that's not breaded and enjoy yourself.

Home-style, country restaurants can be a challenge. But there are usually a few things you can count on. The tricky things can include selections like meat loaf. Our first impression is "Great! That's meat!" But meat loaf is usually made with either oatmeal, crackers or bread in it. So it has hidden carbs. Plus, it's usually served with gravy – always made with flour. And if you're like me, meat loaf just isn't meat loaf without mashed potatoes – another great no-no.

The veggies served with these country meals are often peas, carrots and/or corn too, or something similar – high-carb, comfort foods. If you find yourself horn-swaggled into eating at one of these restaurants, order some kind of a meat dish, like a steak, ham or a pork chop but tell them to hold the gravy, potatoes and bread. Avoid corn, peas and carrots. Summer squash is fine. Indulge in a salad with ranch dressing or vinegar and oil. Order a thick, juicy hamburger (without the bun) or ask if they serve omelets for dinner. That's usually an excellent choice.

Wherever you are, when you order drinks that you want to sweeten, like coffee or tea, there are considerations that are important in choosing which sweetener. Sugar, of course, is the most dangerous to the type II diabetic. Second most dangerous is aspartame, also know as Nutra-Sweet, also known as Equal – the one in the blue packet. It's made of an aspartate molecule, which is toxic to the body, and a phenylalanine molecule, seriously toxic to phenylketoneurics, and bound together by a methyl alcohol molecule, also toxic to the body. There is evidence that all three are released in their toxic forms during the digestion process.

It was also shown in at least one scientific study to be a potent pain-causing substance in a group of Fibromylagia patients. When these patients were taken completely off of all foods and drinks containing aspartame for 4 weeks, all pain symptoms disappeared. When they resumed its use, the pain returned. It's also notorious for causing mood swings and irritability. It's affect on the brain has even been shown to cause weight gain, an ever-present challenge for type II diabetics. Make a real effort to avoid drinks and foods containing this dangerously complicated sweetener. But even this is preferred to sugar for type II diabetics.

Unfortunately, this is probably the most common sweetener in diet soft drinks of all kinds. A few commercial sugar-free drinks are now available with Splenda instead of Nutra Sweet, but you'll seldom find them in restaurants.

Sweet & Low, the sweetener in the pink packet, contains saccharine. Long-term use of saccharine was linked to cancer decades ago, but more recent literature suggests that the dosages at which those tests were administered to the test animals were in massively large doses making the test results unrealistic or at least unreliable when applied to normal human usage. Still, I believe that Sweet & Low or any saccharine sweetener is safer than either Nutra Sweet or Splenda. In restaurants, this is now usually my first choice.

There is a liquid form of Sweet & Low you can buy for home use. The powdered one actually contains other sugar(s). The liquid doesn't. For type II diabetics who are extremely sensitive, this liquid form can make a difference in blood sugar levels.

In the absence of Sweet & Low, I've used Splenda. It's made from a sugar molecule but altered in such a way as to offer the sweetness but not to cause the effects of sugar in the body. There's still research to be done on this one, and some scientific literature has recently been released with warnings about thymus shrinkage which can suppress the immune system. But I still believe it's preferable to using either sugar or aspartame for the diabetic. Splenda is the one in the yellow packet.

My best recommendation for a sweetener is stevia. You won't find it on the restaurant table. You'll need to carry your own. It can be found in most health food stores either in a powdered from or a liquid. The powdered form is usually not pure stevia. It often contains sugars under other names. The powdered form is sometimes tricky to work with because you need so little of it and if too much is used, it can have a bitter component. I personally prefer the liquid form, probably the purest form available as a commercial sweetener. Since you won't find it on the table at restaurants, you'll need to carry your own if stevia is your choice. A small, amber, one-ounce vial is easy to keep in your purse or your pocket. It takes very little to sweeten your drinks, so start with a single drop of the liquid, or enough to cover your little finger nail if you're using the powder, and work up from there to determine how much you personally need to sweeten drinks to your preference.

Some sources also say that stevia can help to actually lower your blood sugar.

When you order coffee in a restaurant, if you use "cream," heavy cream is best, but not often available. Half and half is the next preference. Milk, if you use very little of it, is sometimes acceptable. But you're better off not using any creamer whatsoever if all you have is the powdered type. Made from starchy vegetable sources, they're high in carbs.

As usual, when you're in a restaurant, nearly always avoid the desserts. There are a few exceptions that I know of at the time of this writing. One is the Cheesecake Factory. They make a dessert they call the 6-carb cheesecake, because it has only 6 grams of carbohydrates per slice. It's rich and yummy and very low carb for a true dessert. If you're used to having no desserts but get a chance to try this one, it may even be too much for you. When Linda and I order it, one slice is quite enough to satisfy us both. (Making it the 3-carb dessert!)

Some individually-owned small restaurants around the country are now becoming aware of the low-carb demands for dieters and the huge and growing number of today's type II diabetics. Ask if they offer either carb-free or low-carb desserts. But make sure they're truly low-carb and not the low "NET CARB" desserts that just don't work well for many type II diabetics.

I realize that having the discipline to make the choices outlined in this chapter are often hard when there are so many delicious goodies there just for the ordering or already on your plate and just begging to be lifted onto your fork. The most important thing is that you really do have the opportunity to make the right, healthy choices. The most successful strategy I've ever seen for making the right decisions every time is to make up your mind BEFORE you go into the restaurant or before you leave home to travel. Just allowing yourself to be faced with tough choices as each situation presents itself, without a pre-determined plan, simply places awesome temptation in front of you again and again which can prove insurmountable. It wears a person down like Chinese water torture.

By deciding before you travel or before you eat out, that your choices are going to be the ones that will keep you the healthiest and will be most conducive to extending your life, the more you take those temptations out of your mind completely. The bad choices become items you don't even consider any more and making good choices becomes your ingrained habit.

Either way, you will be forming habits in your food choices. You can be the master of your habits or their slave. The choice is always yours.

A Visit To The Health Food Store

Before I get into the specifics of this chapter, I want to point out that there are two ways of going about trying to re-establish good health. One is "taking stuff." The other way is "corrective actions." The more desirable of the two is the latter. Most of this book addresses taking corrective actions in the form of making proactive, on-going, dietary changes. This chapter, however, addresses "taking stuff" - using the many wonderful foods, vitamins, minerals and herbs that are available at your local health food store for minimizing your diabetes symptoms and preventing them whenever possible. That being said:

The first thing to understand about the supplements you buy at the health food store is that even though they might come in tablets or capsules they're simply not medicines or drugs. They're foods! They put them into tablets and capsules so that you don't have to chew them up and experience the often unpleasant tastes you might find if you consumed them in a straight food form.

Some people may be surprised to read that these "medicinal" supplements with such powerful benefits are just foods but we use many different foods for their specific physical benefits all the time. We drink coffee for its transient energy. We eat chocolate because of the feeling of well-being it produces. We eat turkey or drink chamomile tea for their calming and sleep-promoting qualities. Nearly all foods produce some type of a specific response in our bodies. The foods we find in supplements from the health food stores are relatively pure forms of foods with powerful, individualized effects as well.

We've already discussed some general food categories: carbohydrates, proteins, fats and fiber, fiber not really having nutritive value but offering other benefits. Now let's look at some specifics.

First, let's look at some that have particular benefits for people who suffer from type II diabetes. Vitamin A (Vitamin A palmitate is best) is of special interest because people with diabetes have difficulty converting beta-carotene into vitamin A. Beta carotene is the main food source we use to manufacture our own vitamin A inside our bodies. Beta-carotene comes from red and orange foods like carrots, red peppers, oranges, tomatoes, squash, etc.. Because of the diabetic's inability to make the conversion from beta-carotene to vitamin A easily, getting vitamin A in a state that has already been converted, in a supplement form, is particularly helpful.

Vitamin A is responsible for differentiating cells in the body into their individual specialties. This important process should concern diabetics because of the cellular changes that occur in the blood vessels and because of the need to develop new cells continually within the body's immune system. Some people can double up on their intake of vitamin A palmitate for a few days when they feel a cold or flu coming on and avoid it or minimize the time that they must fight it.

Because vitamin A is the vitamin that's necessary for cell differentiation – in other words, for cells to become specialized into nerve cells, skin cells, heart cells, bone cells, etc. – it also enjoys a well-deserved reputation for being an anti-cancer food. Cancer cells are basically an un-differentiated cell – a cell that doesn't know what it wants to be – an aggressive cell with no specialty.

Vitamin A, however, is one of the few vitamins on which a person can actually overdose. Limit your vitamin A supplements to 50,000 IU's daily. A minimum, daily dose for maintenance would be about 25,000 IU's.

The vitamin B complex is also of particular interest to the diabetic because of its anti-stress qualities. The B complex is vital for proper nerve function, for building red blood cells and for giving you energy and stamina. Niacin, vitamin B3, (dosage as directed on the bottle) is good for keeping the arteries clean and controlling triglycerides but taken by itself, it can produce a "niacin flush," an uncomfortable, hot, red face and ears that lasts for several minutes. So most people prefer to take Niacin in a B complex form. Vitamin B3 also targets insulin resistance, a special goal for the type II diabetic.

Vitamin B12 is the main B vitamin for energy and stamina. It's also a vital component in producing blood cells. Recommended doses for B12 would be at least 250 mcg per day. Vitamin B12, except for a few minor exceptions, is not available from vegetable sources and is almost always obtained from meat. Fortunately, it's one of the vitamins that can be stored in the liver for later use.

Vitamin B6 is especially good for nerve function. It's often recommended for people with carpal tunnel syndrome. It won't stop it, but it will help maintain nerve health or reduce nerve destruction. People who keep a dream journal often find that they can remember their dreams much better when they take a regular vitamin B6 supplement. I like to keep a detailed daily dream journal myself, so I use about 200 to 500 mg of B6 per day as an additional supplement to my B complex.

Vitamins B1 and B6 are also reputed to repel mosquitoes and biting insects when people use them regularly. If you live where the West Nile Virus has been reported, these may be of special interest to you.

The B vitamins are so revitalizing that they're best taken in the morning. For most people, taking them in the late afternoon or evening can keep them from sleeping well.

Vitamin C is vital to life. I'm always amazed when people tell me "I'm allergic to vitamin C." If they truly were, they would be dead! No living animal, including human beings, can survive without vitamin C. It's impossible. If a doctor has told you that you're allergic to vitamin C, there's certainly another factor that's not being addressed and that doctor doesn't understand the vital role of vitamin C in the physiology of all living animals. A person might develop an allergy to a particular SOURCE of vitamin C, but not the vitamin C itself. Manufactured vitamin C (ascorbate / citric acid), for instance, comes from an artificial, non-natural source. Vitamin C from natural sources such as rose hips, acerola cherries, chile peppers, green leafy vegetables, etc., are normally very good sources. Manufactured Vitamin C is not the same as a natural vitamin C, regardless of what your medical doctor, druggist or chemistry Ph.D. tells you. It simply is not the same! There may be allergies to the binders in vitamin C tablets or allergies to components of citrus fruits, but it's certainly not the vitamin C itself. Without vitamin C, life cannot be sustained in mammals (of which we are one).

Vitamin C is particularly important to diabetics because it's so vital to tissue repair - healing. Poor healing is one of the major threats to diabetics. This poor ability to heal is the reason that every day in America, 170 diabetics lose a leg or a foot in the advanced stages of diabetes - more than 62,000 a year! So anything that you can include in your daily intake of foods that will promote healing, you really should have it!

According to Dr. Joel D. Wallach, 1991 Nobel Prize nominee in medicine, and originator of the internationally famous tapes, *"Dead Doctors Don't Lie,"* and *"Dead Doctors Don't Lie II,"* adequate amounts of vitamin C, particularly in combination with bioflavonoids, can also help to prevent the formation of plaque in the arteries – a big concern for diabetics. According to Dr. Wallach, tiny, microscopic "cracks" develop in arteries that are weak and vulnerable. This is further complicated in type II diabetics because, according to Frances Fitzgerald, co-author of *A Woman's Guide to a Healthy Heart*, "as excess insulin pours through the arteries, it damages the arterial lining, increasing the risk of cardiovascular problems."

These tiny cracks in the arteries pose a danger to the blood vessels and their ability to contain the blood within their walls. Cholesterol present in the blood plasma mercifully attaches to these tiny cracks as a means of patching them, kind of like microscopic Band-Aids. Over time, these cholesterol patches, in respose to damage from homocysteine, develop into plaque deposits. But, according Dr. Wallach, when one has an adequate intake of vitamin C (especially with bioflavonoids), it maximizes the strength, elasticity and integrity of the arterial walls. They develop fewer "cracks," sustain less damage and there's no need for the cholesterol to make patches so plaques don't form. According to this explanation, adequate amounts of vitamin C with bioflavonoids can significantly prevent the development of atherosclerosis (arterial plaques).

How much vitamin C is enough? Start at 4 grams (4,000 mg) per day for the average adult. If you smoke, add another 2 grams automatically. Smoking destroys an average of 2,000 mg per day. When you find yourself getting a cold or flu, or other type of illness, increase your daily dose to at least 9 grams per day. If you develop diarrhea at or before you reach this dosage, decrease it by 500 mg per day until the diarrhea stops and maintain that dosage until you're over your illness. The maximum Vitamin C you can take without developing diarrhea is called your "therapeutic dose." When you're over your illness, begin to reduce it by 500 mg per day again until you're back to your baseline of 4,000 mg per day. When you've been taking 9 grams a day for several days, don't just back off all at once. Taper off. That's important.

Taking 500 mg or 1,000 mg of Vitamin C per day is a very minimal dosage. It may be enough to keep you from getting scurvy, the vitamin C deficiency disease that use to kill so many sailors, but it's nowhere nearly enough for optimum health! Nobel Prize winners and nominees have achieved wisdom that is acclaimed by their scientific peers. They agree that vitamin C's one of the most important foods you can swallow!

Vitamin E is also known to be beneficial to the circulatory system – the heart and the blood vessels. This is one of the reasons why it's associated with a great sex life. Of course, circulatory concerns are of great importance to anyone with diabetes.

Vitamin E's anti-oxidant qualities are some of the best of any supplement one can buy. It's best absorbed when combined with selenium. Dr. Julian Whitaker, in his book, *"Dr. Whitaker's Guide to Natural Healing,"* recommends that Type II diabetics take between 1,200 and 1,400 IU's of vitamin E per day.

Pouring the contents of a punctured capsule of vitamin E into your cooking oil when you first open the bottle can also help to reduce the production of free radicals in the oil thus keeping it from becoming rancid.

Chromium GTF (GTF stands for glucose tolerance factor) is an absolutely amazing supplement that should be at the top of the list for every type II diabetic and anybody who wants to control their weight with a low carbohydrate diet. There are many forms of chromium supplements, but my wife and I have found that for type II diabetics specifically, the GTF form seems to work the best.

Chromium is an essential component in carbohydrate metabolism. The minimum daily requirement for chromium is about 90 mcg per day. But the American diet is woefully lacking in this vital mineral. Please keep in mind that 90 mcg is just the level that will keep you from experiencing chromium deficiencies, not enough for optimum health. Three of the most important challenges to diabetics from inadequate chromium are hunger, cravings for carbohydrates and a decreased ability to metabolize carbohydrates.

It often takes a pretty good amount of chromium, especially in the beginning, for people to overcome a chronic chromium deficiency. Supplementing at 90 mcg, then, is not very effective, particularly if you should miss a day here and there. I recommend an absolute minimum of 200 mcg daily just for normal health. But for the type II diabetic or anybody who's adhering to a low carbohydrate regime for any reason, I recommend from 600 to 1,000 mcg per day - 600 mcg as a regular daily supplement and up to 400 mcg as needed to curb cravings.

For instance, it can be beneficial to keep some 200 mcg capsules both at home and where you work to help you with cravings. When you get a case of the "blind, screaming munchies," a craving that just won't leave you alone, just take a capsule and, for most people, the sudden urge to binge will disappear within about 20 minutes. It's a really wonderful tool to help you keep to your healthy eating plan.

In one particular study of both elderly men and elderly women, all with diabetes, chromium supplementation was linked to both an improved glucose tolerance and lower blood fat levels – things one would normally expect from a beneficial increase in the sensitivity to insulin by cells that have developed resistance.

Cinnamon is also a friend to the type II diabetic. It's been shown in studies to help lower blood sugar in type II diabetics. It has insulin-like molecules which appear to make insulin more active so that it can carry the blood glucose into the cells.

A quarter of a teaspoon of cinnamon after each meal is the recommended dose. A word of caution, however, don't mix your cinnamon with sugar to put on your toast! Both the sugar and the toast are basically poison if you're a type II diabetic!

A quarter of a teaspoon of cinnamon in your coffee cup in the mornings can be quite tasty and invigorating. It goes well in many spiced teas too. For convenience, you can purchase cinnamon in your local health food store in tablet or capsule form. My wife, Linda, keeps a bottle of cinnamon tablets in her purse, so it doesn't matter where we are, home, visiting or at a restaurant, she can have her little dose of cinnamon after every meal.

Gymnema sylvestre has long been known to be of great benefit to type II diabetics. The scientific research has demonstrated that Gymnema sylvestre controls blood glucose (blood sugar) by inhibiting glucose uptake in the intestines. It acts as a lipid (fat) lowering agent and may even reduce the incidence of tooth cavities. It also has anti-inflammatory qualities and reduces a person's sensitivity to sweet and bitter tastes. To date there have been no interactions documented and no human toxicity with the plant. Dosage, 400-800 mg/day.

HgH – short for human growth hormone – is an effective supplement to consider as well. I need to qualify that a little, however. If you bought actual human growth hormone, which you certainly can, and legally, you'd be spending a fortune – about $1,500 a month – and you'd be causing your body to produce less and less of its own. The benefits of HgH are tremendous but hardly worth the expense in money and your own, natural, healthy hormone production.

So what most healthcare professionals recommend for HgH supplementation is an HgH stimulator – a spray or an effervescent drink that delivers nutrients which actually cause your body to increase its own natural production of HgH while simultaneously increasing the body's sensitivity to it.

The best way to use HgH is to take it on an empty stomach within a half an hour before going to sleep, then again immediately upon awakening, on a completely empty stomach. To make it maximally effective, make a disciplined effort to perform regular strenuous exercise as we discussed in the chapter on exercise.

You'll find that using HgH increases your energy, increases your ability to do strenuous exercise and, over time, helps you to achieve greater muscle tone. One of the greatest benefits for type II diabetics is the fat-burning action of HgH.

Use HgH daily for two months, then stop for one month, then two months on again, etc. for best results. Taking every third month off keeps your body from becoming desensitized and resistant to it. Dosage indicated on the bottle.

All diabetics should always be concerned about good eye health too, since blindness can be common in the advanced stages. Leutine is a supplement that has specific benefits for the eyes, especially for retinal health. Vitamin A is essential for good night vision. Calcium and magnesium are helpful for micro-circulation in the eyes. Vitamin E is important for strong blood vessels in the eyes. Vitamins A and C and E should be taken in the doses already described.

A supplement called SOD (superoxide dismutase) is known as a great scavenger of free radicals. Free radicals have been implicated in retinal damage, a huge concern for diabetics. Follow directions on the label.

According to some eye doctors who espouse natural means of preventing and treating cataracts (in the earliest stages) glutathione can be quite helpful. Just use as directed on the bottle.

Some years ago, my wife went to the eye doctor for an exam and, during the procedure, they discovered that the pressure in her eyes was high enough to be concerned about glaucoma – 24. The doctor re-scheduled her for another exam in five days to re-check the pressure, stating that if it was still that high, he would give her some prescription eye drops to bring the pressure down.

Linda has very little desire to put her body chemistry out of its natural balance with drugs, even topical ones, so she looked for a better way to bring the pressure down. In her search, she discovered another major benefit of vitamin C with bioflavonoids. She found in Dr. Julian Whitaker's book that I referred to above, that 500 mg of vitamin C with bioflavonoids per kilogram of body weight is a therapeutic dose for working with glaucoma. She simply increased her dosage to 12 grams a day over the next five days, returned for the exam and the doctor was shocked to see that her pressure had dropped to a safe level of 16 in just those five days. Linda, ever the scientist, made sure to verify that the doctor's testing apparatus had been properly calibrated that morning to insure that the test results were valid. So, if glaucoma is a concern for you, consider vitamin C with bioflavonoids at therapeutic doses if you want to stay off the drugs.

Magnesium, especially Magnesium Citrate (which is a little harder to find), should always be on the shopping list for the type II diabetic. Magnesium and calcium must be in a specific balance to maintain good health and carbohydrate metabolism. Many people who experience leg cramps and assume that they're lacking in calcium or potassium are actually missing the balancing effects magnesium. Very few Americans actually lack calcium. Most do lack magnesium.

Magnesium also has a calming effect, so it can help in reducing stress. You've seen in a previous chapter that reducing stress also reduces blood sugar. Of course, if it's calming, it's one of the supplements that's better taken at night before going to bed for better sleep.

Magnesium has been shown to increase insulin sensitivity and in a study of 50 men and women, supplementing with magnesium for 6 months improved blood vessel function and protected the heart. Type II diabetics should use about 1,200 mg per day.

A word about calcium: If you're taking Tums or any other antacid as a calcium source, STOP IMMEDIATELY! Calcium requires an acid environment in the stomach in order for your body to be able to absorb it. An antacid, by definition, causes the acid in your stomach to be neutralized – alkalinized. Because of that, theoretically, regardless of the amount of calcium that may be present in the Tums, your body simply will not be able to absorb it. Not only that, but because you're alkalinizing the stomach, you'll also prevent the digestion of any kind of protein until the stomach can rid itself of any trace of the antacid and re-acidify itself. Review the portion of the Protein chapter regarding combining carbohydrates and proteins to understand how undigested proteins in the body can be toxic.

In addition, a few years ago, there was a scandal about the toxic amounts of lead that were present in popular antacids. Efforts were being made to bring the manufacturers to task about clinging to legal "loopholes" and to bring the lead content of antacids down to "safe" levels. I don't know about you, but to me, there are NO safe levels of lead in anything a human being swallows!

The "purple pills" are also notorious robbers of calcium since they inhibit the body's ability to manufacture stomach acid. However, stomach acid is necessary for absorbing calcium and digesting proteins. In another chapter, I discuss specific alternatives to the purple pills for preventing heartburn and acid reflux.

Milk is another very misunderstood "food" commonly used as a calcium source but that can actually work against you. According to several researchers over the past two decades, homogenized milk undergoes some harmful transformations during the homogenizing process. First, it produces a by-product called Xanthine oxidase, a culprit considered to be a carcinogen (cancer-causing agent). Secondly, as a calcium source, homogenized milk doesn't work well because the homogenizing process also causes the formation of phosphates. These phosphate molecules are so similar to calcium and so electrically active that they bind to the calcium receptor sites in the body and won't let go. When the calcium comes to the receptor sites where it should attach itself, it can't, because the phosphate is already occupying the space and won't give it up for the calcium to bind.

So, drinking homogenized milk from your grocer's shelf can actually prevent you from getting the calcium you need from milk. It also prevents you from getting calcium from any other foods that you eat with it. You can get plenty of calcium from milk if you go outside, milk your own cow and use it without commercial processing. But grocery store milk isn't the same thing at all.

You can get calcium from dairy products that are not made with homogenized milk however – cheese and yogurt for instance.

What's a good source for calcium? Where do cows get theirs? Eating green things! So develop a love for your salads, especially spinach salads, and other dark, green leafy vegetables.

And finally, milk contains lactose, also known as milk sugar - a carbohydrate. The lower the fat content, the more lactose. Skim milk is therefore the highest in milk sugar, heavy cream the lowest.

Zinc is important for many body functions including hair growth, a healthy prostate and resistance to certain infections in the upper respiratory system. Of particular interest to the type II diabetic is the fact that it appears to bind with insulin to enhance its effectiveness and it reduces insulin resistance in the cells. Use 40 to 50 mg per day.

Other foods available at your health food store that can be of specific benefit for the type II diabetic include bitter melon, which is known to be helpful in glucose and fat metabolism; buckwheat seed extracts which reduce blood sugar levels; fenugreek, which helps balance blood sugar and insulin; and garlic, which can lower insulin, blood pressure and triglycerides.

When Linda and I talk with type II diabetics about using supplements from the health food store, typical first reactions are, "Do you mean I need to take all of those supplements every day? That's a lot of pills!" and "That's one or two hundred dollars a month on supplements alone!" Both of these observances are certainly valid. No doubt!

HOWEVER!

Perspective is the fundamental consideration! Even though these supplements are in tablet or capsule form, as we said above, they're foods rather than drugs. So the first thing to do is to change is your mental attitude about it. You're not swallowing dangerous, nasty medicines, you're swallowing *food* that contains life and health! They're basically vital, concentrated groceries rather than medicines. Consider the expense a part of your grocery bill, saving you probably even more money in the area of your medical bills!

If you have trouble swallowing a fistful of supplements at a time, pretend like you're washing down a chewed-up mouthful of your favorite, tasty food with your water and they'll go down a lot easier. Most people have very little difficulty swallowing a mouthful of pie or mashed potatoes. The only difference with a mouthful of supplements is your mental concept of it.

Even then, granted, many people just can't swallow a fistful of supplements all at once. They need to take them one at a time or a few at a time. That's fine. Just be sure you get these healthy supplemental foods that will help you the most and allow you to minimize or even eliminate your need for dangerous, prescription medications – medications that will always produce unwanted side effects! (We know they're dangerous because you have to have a prescription to get them!)

I believe that you're far better off taking a hundred dollars worth of these special foods than you are with taking far more dangerous drugs that are far more expensive anyway. Consider it an investment that will prevent you months and years of feeling really bad and possibly even save you your limbs and/or your eyesight. In addition, even if you pay out a couple hundred dollars a month for supplements, you'll almost certainly save a fortune in what you won't be forking out in doctor bills, even if all you were to pay is deductibles and co-payments, not to mention the fortune that today's typical prescriptions cost! I simply cannot overstate the value of using these supplements daily. It's far less expensive to stay well than it is to get sick and then try to treat it!

Linda, for instance, whose blood sugar was at 485 when she discovered she had diabetes and had had it for some time, injured her leg about a year and a half later. But she had chosen to treat her type II diabetes naturally rather than with drugs during that time. She slipped on some ice, badly scraping her leg and ankle. We were both apprehensive about how her injury might heal since diabetics often have poor healing abilities in the legs and feet. But she had been very disciplined about taking her supplements daily during the whole time she had known about her diabetes. Consequently, she healed remarkably well, and quickly! In fact, she healed faster than many "normally healthy" people! We're both convinced that her regular supplements played a major role in that healing process.

We contend that supplementing is far superior to insurance – that staying well is much better than getting sick and using insurance to pay for doctors, drugs and hospitals. It's that old bit of sage wisdom we've all heard regarding how, "An ounce of prevention is worth a pound of cure."

Again, just consider your supplements as part of your grocery bill since they're necessary foods, not medicines, and learn to do what you need to do to swallow them each and every day. You'll be so glad you did!

When You Just Have
To Have Something Sweet

This has to be one of the greatest stumbling blocks for the majority of type II diabetics and low-carb dieters. If people can't have something sweet from time to time, they tend to just abandon the entire eating strategy. After all, if you can't have a little pleasure in life from time to time, why bother!

In this chapter, you'll see some suggestions for making some really tasty, rich, sweet desserts and other sweet treats, but ones that can be kept well within the limits that the type II diabetic should observe. You'll read about things like meringue cookies and brownies, home-made, low-carb cheesecake, gelato, ice creams of all types, trifles, berry-cream freezes with whipped cream, mock applesauce, café lattes, rich, creamy vanilla tea and more. You don't have to sacrifice great flavors, richness and sweet tasting goodies. You just have to go about it with a slightly different approach.

Even though you can't run down to your local supermarket and pick up these desserts straight from the shelves, the little bit of effort required in preparing them for yourself will be well worth it. In fact, these treats are usually yummy enough to share with your sugar-addicted friends and family members. If you don't tell them that they're eating special, low-carb desserts, they'll usually never know.

Let's start with the simplest "sweet" snacks: Nuts.

Not all nuts are the same, however. All have some carbs. You'll want to avoid relatively high-carb cashews for instance. The trick is to eat the nuts with the fewest carbs and to give up the ones that are high in carbohydrates. In the absence of the high concentrations of carbohydrates in the nuts, the fats in them will not present so many problems, providing the nuts are fresh and not rancid.

Walnuts, are very low in carbohydrates. They're great just plain. They're versatile too. For instance, if you have a dish that calls for a crust, like a quiche or a cheesecake, try replacing the crust with finely chopped walnuts placed in the bottom of a well-buttered pan. If you like, sprinkle a little Sweet & Low or sugar-free caramel Torani syrup over it to add some extra sweetness. A very nice touch, depending on the dish you're making, is to sprinkle some cinnamon on your walnut crust as well. Besides the enhanced flavor, the cinnamon provides the added benefits of helping to lower your blood sugar and being an anti-inflammatory agent!

Another nut well tolerated by many diabetics is almonds. Blue Diamond has a nice variety of almonds to choose from. We keep some on hand all the time. You'll need to experiment with your quantities of each kind of nut and test your resulting blood-sugar levels to determine how much you can indulge yourself with each. My wife, Linda, is very sensitive to even low amounts of carbohydrates; however, she can tolerate a few handfuls of almonds – even smoked almonds – in a single day and does well with chopped walnut crusts on low-carb cheesecake.

Peanuts aren't actually nuts but a sort of pea from the legume family. They aren't nearly as high in carbs as other types of peas though. Some less sensitive type II diabetics can handle limited amounts of peanuts or all-natural peanut butters. CAUTION: Don't use peanut butters like Jif, Peter Pan or other commercial peanut butters that contain added sugar if you're type II diabetic! Laura Scudder and Smuckers have great natural peanut butters that are just peanuts and salt. They're available in both crunchy and smooth.

Look for peanut butters with about a half an inch of oil at the top of the jar. You can either stir the oil into the peanut butter to make it smoother and less dry, or pour it off to keep for other uses.

I have a wooden cutting board for my outdoor kitchen at home and I like to use the peanut oil to oil the board and protect it from the weather. Peanut oil is also great for cooking since it has a high tolerance to heat, reducing the amount of free radicals produced in frying. Adding a little in your home-made ice cream can give it a touch of peanut butter taste too.

For many years, I was a peanut butter and jelly sandwich freak! I would sometimes have two or three of them in a day. Today, instead of peanut butter and jelly sandwiches, I'll take a forkful of peanut butter straight from the jar two or three times a day. It's particularly satisfying when followed up with a nice hot cup of Bigelow's Vanilla tea with a generous portion of heavy cream added and sweetened to taste with Sweet & Low or stevia. You'd be surprised to discover what a rich-tasting treat this can provide when you're haunted by that insatiable urge for a sweet, rich dessert.

A great snack for watching TV is sunflower seeds, straight from the jar. They're not carb-free so you need to experiment to see how many you can consume in a sitting before it has an impact on your blood sugar. But they do seem to be somewhat forgiving. Linda and I sometimes go through a couple of jars in a week. Incidentally, our cat, Mooney, loves them too!

Heavy cream, as I've already mentioned, can actually be a diabetic's greatest friend when it comes to satisfying, rich desserts. But be careful to use regular heavy cream or manufacturer's cream rather than "baker's cream" which has sugar added. Half and half is also higher in lactose (milk sugar), a carbohydrate. The best cream to use is "manufacturers' cream." It usually comes in half-gallons and is found in restaurant supply sources such as Shamrock or Smart & Final. Some manufacturer's cream, like Altadena, contains zero carbs per serving. This is ideal. Others, like Shamrock's, contain only one or less than one gram per serving. You'll need to be a bit more conservative when using these. Cream makes a great dessert just whipped, sweetened and flavored.

Most cheesecake recipes are actually fairly low in carbohydrates if you substitute low-carb sweeteners like stevia or Sweet & Low for sugar and either omit the crust or use a chopped walnut crust like the one mentioned earlier. For fancy flavoring, try small amounts of sugar-free Torani syrups, such as caramel or chocolate. Coffee also provides great flavoring for cheesecakes and homemade ice cream.

Fancy coffees can provide great taste sensations for the dessert lover too. A small, inexpensive cappuccino maker that makes one or two cups at home can give you lots of coffee pleasure.

My favorites are simple lattes (actually "breves"). I like to use gourmet coffees like Starbucks or Gevalia for the richest, fullest flavors. I use a fine, 20-second grind in the coffee holder. With the steam head, I heat and foam heavy cream instead of milk or half and half. It's so much richer and smoother than any café latte you'll ever buy. You'll never want to settle for the regular type again! For an added treat, I'll add some chocolate sugar-free Torani for a mocha or both chocolate and caramel for a "Milky Way mocha." Sweeten to taste with your non-sugar sweetener. Use a little less sweetener than you normally would if you're using the sugar-free Torani syrups because they're sweet too. You'll be a great hit with anyone who has the pleasure of indulging in your fancy coffees!

I'll also use the cappuccino maker to steam a batch of coffee for ice cream. We have a small, home-use ice cream maker that makes enough for about 4 servings. Linda uses regular ice cream recipes but uses non-sugar sweeteners and heavy cream. This creates some texture challenges sometimes because sugar does things to help smooth the texture of normal ice cream, so you have to make some compensations. However, you don't have to compromise!

When making your own ice cream, using heavy cream instead of milk is essential (and a lot tastier). Adding sugar-free gelatin, or an un-flavored gelatin helps to smooth the texture tremendously, often giving it a consistency like gelato. If you've ever been to Italy and experienced this delightful form of ice cream, you'll know exactly what I'm talking about and you'll certainly want to try it.

You can put your own flavors in the ice cream, like steamed coffee (cooled to refrigerator temperature), flavoring extracts, the peanut oil from your natural peanut butter, un-sweetened chocolate, etc., or you can use a sugarless flavored gelatin like cherry or orange. Or make your own combinations like "black forest" using sugar-free cherry gelatin, un-sweetened chocolate and sugar-free chocolate Torani syrup, then topped with whipped cream. Be creative!

Just a short aside: I once thought that steamed coffees, like cappuccinos, had a lot more caffeine than brewed coffee. But it's not true! According to an article on caffeine in the National Geographic in 2004, a cup of brewed coffee has about 200 mg of caffeine as opposed to a steamed coffee which contains an average of only 80 mg. And if you have a problem with caffeine, the gourmet coffee producers all have very nice decaff blends available.

I recommend avoiding the pre-flavored coffees like vanilla, Irish cream, hazelnut, or other similar pre-flavored coffees, and sticking to pure roasted blends like Sumatra, Kona, Ethiopian, etc. to vary the flavor of your coffee. If you want to add other flavors, like vanilla, Irish cream, hazelnut, etc., use the sugar-free Torani syrups to be certain you're avoiding any hidden carbohydrates. It's a lot easier to regulate the intensity of the flavoring this way too. Many of the pre-flavored coffees are what I would consider quite overpowering with their flavorings.

Several companies market very low carbohydrate yogurt desserts that are pretty tasty. By very low carb, I'm talking about 3 grams of actual carbohydrates per serving, not 18 to 21. The only drawback I've experienced with these is that I often want more when I'm done. Linda, on the other hand, is very creative with these things. She can extend one low carb serving of yogurt into satisfying desserts for two people by adding heavy cream, a dash of Torani syrup and a sprinkle of a topping like cinnamon or nutmeg. A little whipped cream helps too. The fat in the cream makes it very satisfying without having to consume unnecessary carbs.

And again, the cream is not actually fattening when used with minimal carbs in the diet. Linda has eliminated more than 85 pounds in 26 months this way!

Another very versatile component of many low-carb desserts that we enjoy is baked meringue. Linda makes a meringue, (see recipes in the cook book, *Joy of Cooking*) sweetened with non-sugar sweeteners then adds flavorings. She then puts dollops of the meringue onto a cookie sheet and bakes them until delicately crisp.

She's used orange flavoring in them, added coconut flavoring and un-sweetened, shredded coconut for macaroons and she's used un-sweetened chocolate, adding her own sweetener. (She's discovered that using both Splenda and stevia together achieves the best sweetening.)

With the chocolate ones, there are two ways to serve the end product. If placed on a plate in the open after baking to a delicate crisp, they make great, very light, chocolate "cookies." If placed into a plastic bag overnight, they develop a more chewy texture, sort of like brownies. They aren't heavy like cookies or brownies, but they are very tasty and fun.

These "cookies" can also contribute to a fun trifle. A trifle is a layered dessert that's usually done with puddings, lady fingers, brandy, fruit and whipped cream. (Many terrors for the type II diabetic!) However, with a few substitutions, you can enjoy trifles to your heart's content. First, in a dessert dish, place one or two softened, sliced meringue "cookies" instead of using the lady fingers. You may want to sprinkle on some rum flavoring or brandy flavoring (but avoid the real thing) to give it an authentic trifle flavor. Next, add about an inch of sugar-free vanilla flavored, home-made custard. Then add either a few thin slices of strawberries, a few blueberries, a few raspberries or blackberries on top of the custard. Add an inch of whipped cream. (For many, the original canned whipped cream – not the low-fat kind – is just fine. It's mostly air and very little carbohydrate so help yourself occasionally.) Then repeat the process a second time in the same dish, top with a large dollop of whipped cream and garnish with a slice of strawberry, a raspberry, blueberry or blackberry. Yummy!

Custards using sugar substitutes are naturally low in carbohydrates and high in protein because of the egg content. The only food more complete than eggs is mothers' milk! Enjoy custards any way you want them. Just use non-sugar sweetening agents.

When you want a nice, cold, wet treat on a hot summer day, try a freezie. All you need is a blender, some ice, your favorite flavoring, some heavy cream, whipped cream, sweetener and a tiny bit of frozen berries of any kind (not pre-sweetened). Blend all the ingredients together. Pour into a glass, top with whipped cream, add about a teaspoon of blueberries, a few slices of a strawberry or a few black cherries and voila! A mighty tasty fruit freezie! For variations include a little sugar-free Jell-O for a smoother, thicker freezie with a fruitier taste.

Earlier in this chapter, I mentioned using gelatin in your home-made ice cream too, to help produce an ideal, creamy texture. Sugar-free gelatin in itself is a great dessert for the type II diabetic. I don't recommend putting fruit in it unless you just add a teaspoon or less of fruit to your bowl of Jell-O just as it's being served. Adding heavy cream to Jell-O, and/or topping it with whipped cream is a delightful touch, however, that fits well with the low-carb diet adding truly satisfying richness for the dessert lover. But be aware that the sugar-free gelatins do contain aspartame and use them sparingly.

Recently, Linda created a mock applesauce that I'd have never realized was not real applesauce if I hadn't known for certain that she would never eat the real thing. Instead of apples, she used a zucchini from our garden that had grown huge! She peeled it, steamed it, put it into a blender with lemon juice, lemon zest, sweetener, cinnamon, nutmeg, a tiny touch of ginger and a dash of sugar-free Torani French vanilla syrup. The texture, appearance, taste and aroma were exactly like applesauce! We were delightedly amazed! Of course, to enjoy it even more, we added a little heavy cream and nutmeg just before serving.

There are definitely certain foods you'll have to exclude from your life on a permanent basis as a type II diabetic if you want to control your diabetes without medications or to control it more effectively in tandem with your medications. But you absolutely don't have to categorically give up wonderful, sweet, rich desserts. You just need to decide that you'll make them all yourself (far tastier than any commercially prepared stuff you can buy anyway), and make them with a new set of guidelines.

We serve these fun treats to our visitors who always "ooh" and "aah" about how great they are. The most common two questions we get about them are "what about all the cream" which is actually fine since the desserts are consumed WITHOUT the carbs; and the second question is, "Can I get the recipe?"

Feeling trapped in self denial is the one major thing that will influence a person the most into abandoning healthy habits. And it's not necessary at all. Simply become familiar with the things you *can* have and focus on them. Then develop a sharp awareness of the things you should avoid and be creative from there. You can do a lot with cream, eggs, sweeteners and a few walnuts, for instance. When you look at a recipe in a magazine or a cookbook, use your imagination to explore how you might substitute the ingredients you CAN have for the ones you should avoid. Just because a recipe calls for sugar and milk chocolate doesn't mean you can't use the recipe. See if you can substitute Sweet & Low and Torani sugar-free chocolate or un-sweetened chocolate. Be disciplined, but be bold!

There are other things you can do in the way of substitution as well. Although not actually a "sweet dish," potato salad can be made very nicely, and with similar flavors, by substituting steamed cauliflower for the potatoes. The same can be done for a mashed potato substitute too. Mash the cooked cauliflower with butter, heavy cream and/or sour cream, and some garlic, just as you would a great mashed potato recipe.

If you think you might be able to use one thing for a substitute, but are unsure of its carbohydrate content, look at the chart in the last chapter of this book or better yet, buy a carbohydrate counter book that's more complete. Once you try a new creation and you decide you like it, be sure to test yourself after eating it to make sure that your body will tolerate it, or if you need to place limits on your consumption.

Being nice to yourself if you have a sweet tooth is the only way to prevent falling off the wagon. And for the type II diabetic, the dietary suggestions in this book should be adopted as a *permanent lifestyle*, not just a temporary, remedial "diet." The next book in this series will be a cookbook. Watch for it.

When The Experts Speak

The major intention of this book was to give you the most basic, most important cornerstones of understanding type II diabetes and suggesting what you might do when the "experts" speak, in the news, in newspaper and magazine articles, on tapes and in lectures, even face-to-face in doctors' offices and in other professionals' offices, you won't have to just take what they're saying at face value as if it were absolute, unquestionable, "gospel" truth.

For instance, as I was proof-reading this manuscript and doing my final re-writes, my wife showed me an article in our local newspaper on the harmful effects of alloxan, a substance used in processing white flour. The article stated that the presence of the alloxan causes physical harm to the beta cells of the pancreas causing them to lose their ability to produce sufficient amounts of insulin. The next thing they said was that this in turn causes adult onset, *type II diabetes.* WRONG! Hopefully, by now you've read enough information throughout this book to know beyond any shadow of a doubt that if something causes a DECREASE in insulin output from the pancreas it absolutely would NOT cause type II diabetes! It would cause *type I diabetes!* Not maybe. Not probably. But absolutely. No question! By definition, type I is an insulin *deficiency.* Type II is an *overabundance* of insulin that results in cells that are resistant to insulin!

Even though the information was important to know, and it's another very important reason for avoiding white bread and anything else made from white flour, the casual, uninformed and consequently misleading declaration that it produces type II diabetes is absolutely,100% wrong and contributes significantly to the massive body of confused misinformation that circulates throughout today's media about type II diabetes.

On January 27th, 2006, Fox News aired an announcement about Exubera, a new, inhalant-spray form of insulin. Every time I saw the announcement and the subsequent commentary, it was praised as a breakthrough for "diabetics," as if all diabetics are the same. I truly hope that you know differently by now from the contents of this book. If it's an insulin product for diabetics, which diabetics would it benefit? It may be fine for the type I but it would contribute to more problems for the type II.

I cannot over-emphasize how important it is to know the distinct and vital differences between type I and type II. Why? Because the way you treat them is extremely different! Treating type II with strategies for type I is dangerous and actually makes the type II diabetes even worse!

After you've finished this book, I strongly urge you to re-read the chapter on contrasting type I diabetes from type II. It's imperative that you fully understand how type II diabetes develops and the relationship of blood sugar, carbohydrates and insulin if you hope to have any chance whatsoever of sorting out all of the old wives tales, masquerading as valid medical information, from what the realities are. I want you to completely understand that type II diabetes is your body's loss of an ability to properly metabolize carbohydrates, even though your body still turns all of your nutrients into blood sugar.

Your body's first choice is to use carbohydrates as fuel. When they're restricted, your body resorts to using fats as its fuel. If both carbs and fats are unavailable, your body will resort to using protein for its glucose source. It is the fact that your body DOES turn everything into blood sugar that is the reason why eating carbohydrates directly as a food group is not necessary.

It's because type II diabetes is your body's inability to properly metabolize carbohydrates that makes it insane to suggest that type II diabetics consume five or six servings of carbohydrates daily; or even one serving for that matter. I agree that it is very difficult, if not impossible, to eliminate all carbohydrates from the daily diet; however, since type II diabetes is fundamentally caused from long-term "abuse," whether intentionally or unknowingly as a victim of the standard, high-carb, American diet; and yo-yo dieting; once you've determined that you're a type II diabetic, eliminating as many carbs from your diet as you can is the only sane and rational approach to controlling it.

If you were allergic to strawberries, you wouldn't eat strawberries. If you choked on cottage cheese, you wouldn't eat cottage cheese. When your body can't handle sudden and drastic reactions to carbohydrates, it's simply not healthy, or even reasonable, to consume them.

It's vital that you understand that unlike type I diabetes which is the result of a disease process, type II diabetes is actually a survival mechanism that has gone too far and set your entire carbohydrate metabolism completely out of balance. The difference between these two types of diabetes represents a chasm that few healthcare professionals today seem to fully grasp. And the victims of these shortcomings are the unsuspecting type II diabetics taking the less-than-sound advice of these well-meaning but un-enlightened "experts."

So, if you're reading an article which suggests that you eat some kind of food that contains carbohydrates, claiming that it will "help your diabetes," you must first understand that the author probably has no idea of what type II diabetes actually is, how it develops, how it differs from type I diabetes, or the very real dangers of contributing to its continued development with the exact agent that is its very cause.

I see ads on TV suggesting that diabetics (not mentioning whether they're addressing type I, type II or all diabetics) drink preparations like Glucerna (weight-loss shakes) or Ensure (a generic food substitute) with the assumption that losing weight will be the result and that losing weight will reduce your diabetic symptoms and risks.

First, please remember that this thinking is actually backward. The extra weight is the RESULT of the pre-diabetic and type II diabetic condition, not the CAUSE. Secondly, those drinks are typically very high in carbohydrates (poison for the type II diabetic). And third, the low fat diet (which these drinks represent) has been proven to be an exercise in futility for America. Over the past few decades in which the low-fat diet has been increasingly recommended and practiced, the average weight of the American adult has increased by from 10 to 20 pounds, depending on the study you read, and obesity has become an epidemic of major proportion throughout the population at large.

From time to time, articles and news bytes appear stating that a certain kind of food is "good for diabetics" (again without qualifying for which type). We've seen many of these – articles that praise the benefits of whole grain breads, for instance, because it's high in fiber. But they're still grains and high in carbohydrates. Not only do the carbs increase your blood sugar, they increase serum cholesterol, as you read earlier, because of its stimulation of insulin and insulin's direct effect on how cells produce and use cholesterol. Controlling cholesterol (180 to 200mg/dl) is a common concern for the type II diabetic because of cardiovascular health concerns.

My wife and I read one article stating that bananas are particularly good for diabetics. Linda tried it. It shot her blood sugar sky high and she was sick for three days as a direct result of taking that advice at face value. Her physical response was logical because bananas are one of the fruits that are exceptionally high in carbs. She's had similar reactions with other carb-containing foods and supplements that were supposed to have beneficial effects for "the diabetic." Be aware that, as stated earlier, each person is different in how his or her body reacts to carbohydrates, and that a disproportionately large percentage of healthcare professionals don't understand the important contrasts between type I and type II diabetes.

Authors, who are looking to sell their articles with some sort of "secret" piece of "magical" information as their selling point, as often as not, don't have the background to see the whole picture in terms of human physiology and pathological processes, especially regarding type II diabetes. Regardless of how reasonable the article might initially appear, the author's credentials don't always assure true qualifications.

Ideally, if you're a type II diabetic, you're going to want to keep your carbohydrate count to 30 grams or less per day. If you're an exceptionally sensitive type II diabetic, you'll want to keep it below 20 grams.

If you're a type I diabetic, the kind that results from the pancreas failing to produce insulin, often called juvenile onset diabetes or JOD, it's a little different. The carbohydrates themselves haven't caused your diabetes to manifest, as in type II, but you still have to regulate your blood sugar because of the lack of insulin production to take the blood sugar out of your blood and into the cells. If the glucose can't get out of your blood and into your cells, it causes all of the symptoms and dangers associated with hyperglycemia (high blood sugar). For the type I diabetic, the concern is acquiring insulin from outside sources then administering it in the right proportions to take the blood sugar sufficiently into the cells but without decreasing the blood sugar to abnormally and dangerously low levels. This is typically something of a balancing act and must be worked out differently for each type I diabetic.

There is a tendency for patients, doctors and other well-meaning advisors to confuse the two types of diabetes; however, this is incredibly dangerous because they are so opposite, even though they have identical symptoms. You must always be acutely aware of the differences because any information you receive about diabetes must necessarily be weighed in light of these differences. You are ultimately the one who has to determine whether the person disseminating that information, doctor or otherwise, actually knows the difference between the two and how important that distinction is. Your advisors may mean well and truly believe what they are telling you, but if they aren't aware of the extremely important differences between these two types of diabetes, they can hurt you, or more importantly, they can cause you to hurt yourself!

There's a saying in the financial markets that goes, "Nobody cares about your money like you do," meaning that leaving your financial decisions to others carries certain risks regardless of that person's credentials. It's true. It's also true that nobody cares about your health like you do. People are free and easy with their advice because it's not their own bodies and they won't have to physically live with the results of their advice, or die from it themselves. Make sure you know how to evaluate information that people give you about diabetes, especially type II diabetes, by knowing what diabetes is, how both types develop and what is most dangerous to those who have it.

Another saying in the financial markets is, "Nobody knows what you think they know," meaning that you're usually better off doing your own research and making your financial investments based on your own knowledge of the basics. The same is true of your health. Nobody knows what you think they do. Your best bet is to know all you can about your own condition, to know how to test for real-time numbers, to understand the significance of the measurements of your own health status and especially to make your own decisions based on your own knowledge of the basics.

Blindly putting our faith into healthcare professionals, nutritionists and hospitals can be as dangerous as blindly following the advice of newspaper and magazine articles. According to an article that appeared in the <u>AARP Bulletin</u> in the summer of 2005, over 90,000 people die *unnecessarily* in American hospitals every year. My point is that unsubstantiated trust in anyone just because he or she has a specific title (like "doctor" or "nurse" or "nutritionist") can actually prove to be lethal, and according to existing records, often is.

Never take what anyone tells you just at face value without some criteria for determining whether it will be true for you as an individual in your own personal circumstances. The best way to do that is to prove or disprove the information by testing your own urine and blood for glucose content. If you want to test a food you read about, eat it sparingly, then test your urine and/or your blood throughout the day to see if it works for you as an individual the way it's supposed to work according to the person who recommended it. In 20 years plus as a doctor, I've learned that my professor was right when he said, "People's bodies don't read the books!" There's always someone who doesn't fit the neat little boxes into which the statisticians want to categorize people. If you're one of those people whose body works differently than the majority of others' do, it will matter very little to you how everybody else's bodies work, but rather, only how your own does.

Read what you can, then prove it to yourself or disprove it by testing your own body's responses. This includes the information you've read in this book. Test my information with the same, tough scrutiny. The tests you do on your own body will tell you how true this information is for you, specifically. Any information meant for the type II diabetic must absolutely work for you as a unique individual or it has no value for you – no practical truth.

One of the very best ways to discover exactly what those truths are for your own body is to keep a <u>Food and Testing Journal</u>. Pick up a diary-type book at any stationary store for writing your journal. Make records each day, especially for the first few months to a year.

On each page, draw a vertical line down the center of the page. Each page will represent one day. Put the date at the top of each page. To the left of your line, write down each item you eat or drink on that day. Include everything: snacks, salad dressings, condiments, meals and what you drink, even water. On the right side of that line write all of your test results for that day (see the chapter on testing) and how you felt after eating or drinking those items. Note sensations like dizziness, crabbiness, fatigue, energetic feelings, feeling clear-headed, hunger, cravings – anything you notice. Review your journal often.

After a while, patterns will emerge to demonstrate for you how long it takes for the effects of foods to show up in your blood and urine, exactly what foods set you out of balance the most, what you handle the best, and who is right and who is not so right in their recommendations for what you should or should not be eating as a type II diabetic. After you've established your own patterns and have become familiar with them, you'll become more and more able to determine whether that new "expert" has valid advice or not, even before you try it! You'll be able to see the results of your own experiments with their recommendations, positive or negative, usually within hours. You'll never again be in a quandary about whose advice you should heed. You'll know beyond any doubt whatsoever, that the only advice that will ever be valid for you will come from the results of the testing that you do on your own body. Through experimenting with what you eat and subsequent testing, your own body will be your most useful and trustworthy advisor.

When the "experts" speak, certainly keep an open mind, but be sure to filter each and every bit of their information through your own knowledge and testing procedures. It may surprise you to discover that, quite often, you'll be more knowledgeable than they are on the subject of type II diabetes.

Abbreviated Nutrition Chart

Although I suggest that you go out and find a good carbohydrate counter book at your local book store, I wanted to include a basic chart for you in the mean time. The following chart, adapted from "Joy of Cooking," lists some foods, their serving sizes, and their contents of carbohydrates, protein, fats, and fiber, in grams per serving. Please keep in mind that the most important of these, the one that you need to watch the closest is the carbohydrate count.

Food	Serving size	Carbs	Protein	Fat	Fiber
Almonds, raw	1 cup	28	27	71	15
Apple, raw	1 small	21	0	1	4
Apple juice	1cup	29	0	0	2
Apricot	3	12	1	0	3
Artichoke	1 whole	10	4	1	5
Asparagus	1 cup	6	3	0	3
Avocado	1/2 cup	9	2	18	6
Bacon	1 slice	0	2	3	0
Banana	1	27	1	1	3
Barley	1 cup	135	23	4	32
Baked beans	1 cup	52	12	1	13
Beans, green	1 cup	10	2	0	4
Beans, kidney	1 cup	40	15	1	13
Beans, lima	1 cup	42	15	1	14
Beans, navy	1 cup	19	7	0	4

Bean sprouts	1 cup	**6**	3	0	2
Beef, dried	3 oz	**1**	25	3	0
Beef, lean ground	3 oz	**0**	15	18	0
Beef, roast	3 oz	**0**	25	6	0
Beef, tongue	3 oz	**19**	18	0	0
Beer	12 oz	**13**	1	0	1
Beets, chopped	1 cup	**24**	4	0	8
Blackberries	1 cup	**18**	1	1	8
Blueberries	1 cup	**21**	1	1	4
Bologna	1 slice	**1**	3	8	0
Chicken bouillon	1 cube	**1**	0	0	0
Bran, oat	1 cup	**4**	15	5	13
Braunschweiger	1 oz	**1**	4	9	0
Brazil nuts	1 cup	**18**	20	93	8
Bread, white	1 slice	**12**	2	1	2
Bread, whole wheat	1 slice	**12**	2	1	2
Broccoli, raw	1 cup	**5**	3	0	3
Brussel sprouts	1 cup	**18**	7	1	8
Butter, salted	1 tsp.	**0**	0	4	0
Butter, unsalted	1 tsp.	**tr.**	0	4	0
Cabbage	1 cup	**4**	1	0	2
Cake, angel food	2 oz slice	**33**	3	0	1
Cake, pound	2 oz slice	**28**	3	11	0

Cantaloupe	1 large	**98**	11	1	14
Caramels	2	**10**	0	0	0
Carrots	1 cup	**16**	2	0	5
Cashews	1 cup	**45**	21	64	4
Cauliflower	1 cup	**5**	2	1	3
Celery	2 stalks	**3**	1	0	1
Cheese, American	1 oz	**0**	6	9	0
Cheese, Cheddar	1 oz	**0**	7	9	0
Cheese, cottage	1 cup	**3**	25	1	0
Cheese, Parmesan	1 Tbsp	**0**	2	2	0
Cheese, ricotta	1 cup	**12**	28	14	0
Cheese, Roquefort	1 oz	**1**	6	9	0
Cheese, Swiss	1 oz	**1**	8	8	0
Cherries	15	**17**	1	1	2
Chicken, dark meat	3.5 oz	**0**	27	10	0
Chicken, breast, fried	1	**1**	58	8	1
Chocolate, bittersweet	1oz	**16**	2	10	2
Chocolate, milk	1 oz	**16**	2	9	1
Chocolate, fudge	1 piece	**14**	0	1	0
Chocolate, syrup	1 Tbsp	**12**	0	0	1
Clams	3 oz	**2**	11	1	0

Coconut	1 cup	**12**	3	27	7
Cod	3 oz	**0**	19	1	0
Coffee	1 cup	**1**	0	0	0
Corn	1 ear	**19**	3	1	2
Corn flakes	1 cup	**26**	2	0	1
Cornmeal	1 cup	**26**	3	1	2
Cornstarch	1 cup	**117**	0	0	1
Corn syrup	1 oz	**23**	0	0	0
Crab meat	4 oz	**0**	21	1	0
Cracker, Graham	1	**5**	0	1	0
Cracker, Saltine	1	**2**	0	0	0
Cranberries	1 cup	**14**	0	0	5
Cream, heavy	1Tbsp	**1**	0		0
Cream, whipped	1 Tbsp	**1**	0	1	0
Cucumber	1 cup	**3**	1	0	1
Dates	3	**19**	1	0	2
Doughnut, glazed	1	**23**	2	10	1
Dressing, 1,000 Island	1 Tbsp	**2**	0	6	0
Dressing, French	1 Tbsp	**3**	0	6	0
Duck, roasted	1	**0**	104	50	0
Egg, poached	1	**1**	6	5	0
Egg, white	1	**0**	4	0	0
Egg, yolk	1	**0**	3	5	0

Eggplant	1 cup	**5**	1	0	2
Endive	1 cup	**2**	1	0	2
English muffin	1	**26**	4	1	2
Fig, fresh	1	**10**	0	0	2
Flour, cake	1 cup	**85**	9	1	2
Flour, rye	1 cup	**0**	29	12	0
Flour, whole wheat	1 cup	**87**	16	2	15
Flour, white, all-purpose	1 cup	**88**	12	1	3
Flounder	3-4 oz	**0**	21	5	0
Frankfurter, beef/pork	1	**1**	6	17	0
Gelatin, plain, sugared	1 cup	**34**	4	0	0
Gin	4 oz	**0**	0	0	0
Ginger ale, sugared	12 oz	**32**	0	0	0
Goose, wild, roasted	4 oz	**0**	28	25	0
Grape juice	1 cup	**38**	1	0	0
Grapefruit	1	**29**	3	1	18
Grapefruit juice, un-sweetened	1 cup	**22**	1	0	0
Grapes, green, seedless	1 cup	**16**	1	0	1
Grits	1 cup	**32**	3	0	0

Half and half	1 cup	1	0	2	0
Halibut, broiled	3 oz	0	23	3	0
Ham, lean, roasted	3 oz	0	21	5	0
Herring	3 oz	0	15	8	0
Herring, pickled	1 piece	5	7	9	0
Hollandaise sauce	1 Tbsp	5	7	9	0
Honey	1 Tbsp	17	0	0	0
Honeydew melon	1 cup	16	1	0	1
Horseradish	1 Tbsp	3	0	0	0
Ice cream, regular, vanilla	1 cup	19	4	11	0
Icing	1 cup	75	1	0	0
Jam	1 Tbsp	13	0	0	0
Kale	1 cup	7	2	1	3
Ketchup	4 oz	4	0	0	0
Kiwi	1	11	0	0	3
Lamb chops	3 oz	0	30	12	0
Lard	1 Tbsp	0	0	13	0
Leek	1	12	1	0	5
Lentils	1 oz	17	5	0	5
Lettuce, iceberg	1 head	21	6	1	9
Lime	1	7	0	0	2
Liver (beef)	4 oz	7	23	4	0

Liverwurst	1 slice	**0**	3	5	0
Lobster	1 cup	**1**	43	2	0
Macaroni	1 cup	**32**	5	1	2
Maple syrup	1 Tbsp	**12**	0	0	0
Margarine (corn oil)	1 tsp	**0**	0	4	0
Marmalade	1 oz	**17**	0	0	0
Marshmallows	5	**29**	1	0	0
Mayonnaise	1 Tbsp	**0**	0	11	0
Melba toast	1 slice	**3**	1	0	0
Milk (buttermilk)	1 cup	**13**	4	0	7
Milk, 1%	1 cup	**12**	8	3	0
Milk, 2%	1 cup	**12**	8	5	0
Milk, chocolate	1 cup	**26**	7	7	1
Milk, skim	1 cup	**12**	8	0	0
Milk, whole	1 cup	**11**	8	8	0
Molasses	1 Tbsp	**11**	0	0	0
Muffin, corn	1	**29**	3	5	2
Mushrooms	1 cup	**3**	1	0	1
Mustard greens	1 cup	**3**	3	0	3
Nectarine	1	**16**	1	1	2
Noodles, egg	1 cup	**40**	8	2	2
Oatmeal	1 cup	**25**	6	2	4
Okra, boiled	1 cup	**7**	2	0	3

Oil, corn	1 Tbsp	**0**	0	14	0
Oil, olive	1 Tbsp	**0**	0	14	0
Oil, peanut	1 Tbsp	**0**	0	14	0
Oil, Safflower	1 Tbsp	**0**	0	14	0
Oil, sesame	1 Tbsp	**0**	0	14	0
Olives, black or green	1 large	**1**	0	1	0
Onion, raw	1 cup	**14**	2	0	3
Orange	1	**15**	1	0	3
Orange juice	1 cup	**26**	2	1	1
Oysters, raw	1 cup	**13**	12	4	0
Parsley	1 cup	**0**	0	0	0
Parsnips	1 cup	**27**	2	0	6
Peach	1	**10**	1	0	2
Peanuts, unsalted	1 cup	**31**	35	73	12
Pear	1	**25**	1	1	4
Peas	1 cup	**25**	9	0	9
Peas, black-eyed	1 cup	**100**	39	2	18
Pecans	1 cup	**18**	8	78	7
Pepper, green	1	**5**	2	0	3
Pepperoni	1 slice	**0**	1	2	0
Persimmon	1	**8**	0	0	
Pickle, large dill	1	**8**	0	0	0
Pineapple	1 cup	**19**	1	1	2

Plum	1 cup	**38**	2	2	4
Pomegranate	1	**26**	1	0	1
Popcorn (popped)	1 cup	**8**	1	1	1
Pork (lean)	4 oz	**0**	32	5	0
Potato, baked	2.9 oz	**51**	5	0	5
Potato, boiled	1 cup	**49**	5	0	4
Preserves	1 Tbsp	**13**	0	0	0
Pretzels, thin stick	5	**1**	0	0	0
Prunes, dried	1 cup	**88**	4	1	10
Pumpkin	1 cup	**8**	1	0	1
Rabbit, roasted	4 oz	**0**	25	7	0
Radishes	3	**0**	0	0	0
Raisins	1 cup	**115**	5	1	6
Raisin Bran	1 cup	**43**	5	1	7
Raspberries	1 cup	**14**	1	1	8
Red snapper, baked	3 oz	**0**	22	1	0
Rice, brown, cooked	1 cup	**46**	5	2	4
Rice, white, cooked	1 cup	**53**	4	0	1
Rice, wild, cooked	1 cup	**35**	7	1	3
Roll, hard, white	2 oz	**30**	6	2	1
Root beer	12 oz	**39**	0	0	0
Salami	1 slice	**0**	6	10	0

Salmon, broiled	3 oz	0	29	15	0
Sardines, in oil	3 oz	0	21	10	0
Sauerkraut	1 cup	4	0	0	4
Sausage, pork, link	1	0	3	4	0
Scallop	1 large	1	5	0	0
Seeds, pumpkin	1 oz	4	7	16	0
Seeds, sunflower	1 oz	5	6	14	3
Sherbet	1 cup	59	2	4	0
Sherry, dry	4 oz	9	0	0	0
Shrimp, boiled	3 oz	0	18	1	0
Sole	3 oz	0	18	1	0
Spaghetti, plain, cooked	1 cup	40	7	1	2
Spareribs, roasted	3 oz	0	24	12	0
Spinach, raw	1 cup	2	2	0	2
Squash, butternut, baked	1 cup	8	1	0	3
Strawberries	1 cup	11	1	0	3
Sugar, brown	1 cup	214	0	0	0
Sugar, white	1 cup	200	0	0	0
Swordfish, broiled	3 oz	0	22	4	0
Taco shell, baked	1	8	1	3	1
Tangerine	1	9	0	0	2
Tartar sauce	1 Tbsp	1	0	8	0

Tea, un-sweetened	1 cup	**0**	0	0	0
Tofu, firm	8 oz	**10**	36	20	5
Tofu, soft	8 oz	**5**	11	7	0
Tomato, ripe, raw	1	**6**	1	0	1
Tomato juice	1 cup	**10**	2	0	2
Tomatoes, canned	1 cup	**11**	2	0	2
Tortilla, corn	1	**12**	1	1	1
Trout, broiled	4 oz	**0**	24	11	0
Tuna, canned in water	0	**29**	1	0	0
Turkey	5 oz	**6**	5	0	0
Turnips, boiled	1 cup	**11**	2	0	4
Vanilla extract	1 Tbsp	**4**	0	0	0
Veal, lean, roasted	3 oz	**0**	22	5	0
Venison, baked	1 pound	**0**	103	11	0
Vienna sausage	1	**0**	2	4	0
Vodka	4 oz	**0**	0	0	0
Walnuts, chopped	1 cup	**15**	30	71	6
Watercress, chopped	1 cup	**0**	1	0	1
Watermelon	1 cup	**12**	1	1	1
Wheat germ	1 Tbsp	**4**	2	1	1
Whiskey	4 oz	**0**	0	0	0
Whitefish, broiled	3 oz	**0**	21	6	0

Wine, dry, red	4 oz	**1**	0	0	0
Yams, baked	1 cup	**38**	2	0	5
Yogurt, full-fat, plain	1 cup	**11**	7	2	0
Yogurt, non-fat, plain	1 cup	**19**	13	0	0
Zucchini, boiled	1 cup	**7**	1	0	3

Use this chart to look up your favorite foods and, if you need to change your eating habits, look up the carbohydrate contents of the new foods you are considering. As many foods as there are listed in this chart, however, there are certainly many that are not. That's why buying a separate book with a more complete chart can be of particular help to you.

Index

I

India 6
Insulin shock 3
Italian food 103

J

Jell-O 86, 102, 131
JOD 4, 139
Journal of the AMA xii

K

Ketodiastix 91
Ketostix 16, 17, 29, 91

L

LDL's 22–25, 27, 29
Leutine 118
Lobelia 69, 70
Low fat diet 24, 138
Lymphatic system 59, 60

M

Magnesium 70, 118–120
Maltodextrin 7
Mannitol 7
Mannose 7
Manufacturers cream 127
McDonald's 78, 106
Meditation 73
Melatonin 70, 71
Meringue cookies 86, 100, 125
Mexican food 101, 102
Milk 29, 85, 88, 102, 104, 106, 120,
        121, 127, 128, 131, 132, 145
Milky Way mocha 106, 128
Mitochondria 62

N

Net Carbs 47–50, 53, 99
Neurotransmitters 20
Niacin 113
Nutritionists xix, xx, xxi, 47, 140

Nuts xii, 47, 50, 55, 85, 126, 144

O

Obesity 12, 26, 57, 77, 83, 86, 138
Osteoarthritis 57
Osteoporosis 58

P

PABA 59
Pancreas 1–4, 9, 10, 11, 13, 26, 54,
        135, 139
Peanut butter 127, 129
Phosphates 121
Pitting edema 61
Polydypsia 1, 13
Polyphasia 1, 13
Polyuria 1, 13
Power nap 68
Pre-diabetic xviii, 11, 12, 39, 54, 92,
        97–99, 138
Progesterone 20, 58
Protein Power xx, 30
Purple pills 37, 40, 41, 120
Pyloric valve 38

R

Real Animal Way 79
Rheumatoid Arthritis 25
Rolaids 37

S

Seafood 85, 102, 103, 106
Sleeping pills 71
Sleep Number Beds 75
Snoring xxi
Statin drugs 25
Steak houses 102
Subway 104
Sugar curing 4
Sunflower seeds 127
Super oxide dismutase (SOD) 118

T

Tempurpedic beds 74, 75
Testosterone 20
Thai food 105
Thirst, constant 1
Tryptophan 71
Tums 37, 41, 120

U

Urination, frequent 69, 73

V

Valerian 69
Vegetarians 33
Venous thrombosis 62
Vietnamese food 105
Vitamin A 112, 118
Vitamin B12 35, 41, 57
Vitamin B3 113
Vitamin B6 113
Vitamin B complex 113
Vitamin C 113–115
vitamin D 58, 59
Vitamin E 115, 116, 118

W

Weight loss xxi, 3, 17, 30, 64
Wendy's 104
West Nile Virus 113
Wolfe's Law 58, 59

X

Xanthene oxidase 121
Xylitol 7

Z

Zinc 121